1983

THE DEFINITION OF QUALITY AND APPROACHES TO ITS ASSESSMENT

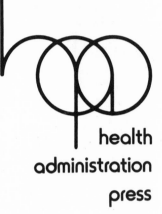

health
administration
press

EXPLORATIONS IN QUALITY ASSESSMENT AND MONITORING

Volume I

THE DEFINITION OF QUALITY AND APPROACHES TO ITS ASSESSMENT

Avedis Donabedian, M. D., M. P. H.
The University of Michigan

Health Administration Press
Ann Arbor, Michigan

1980

Library of Congress Cataloging in Publication Data

Donabedian, Avedis.
   The definition of quality and approaches to its
assessment.

   (His Explorations in quality assessment and
monitoring; pt. 1)
   Includes bibliographies and indexes.
   1. Medical care—Evaluation. 2. Medicine—
Philosophy.   I. Title. [DNLM: 1. Quality
assurance, Health care. 2. Evaluation studies.
W84.1 D674e]
RA399.A1D65   pt. 1   362.1′068s [362.1′068]
80–15173
ISBN 0–914904–47–7
ISBN 0–914904–48–5 (pbk.)

   This volume is based on work supported by the National Center
for Health Services Research under grants 1-R01-HS-02081-01,
5-R01-HS-02081-02, 2-R01-HS-02081-03, and 3-R01-HS-02081-
02S1. The views expressed in it are those of the author alone, and
do not in any way represent the National Center.

Health Administration Press
School of Public Health
University of Michigan
Ann Arbor, Michigan 48109

313–764–1380

DEDICATION

I have written this book in memory of
SAMUEL DONABEDIAN
my father
and a good physician
for love of whom I have loved in medicine
all that is good, and hated
all that is less than perfect
and of
MARITZA DONABEDIAN
my mother
who taught me how to love and how to hate
but, above all, to endure

Table of Contents

Preface

With this small book I take another step forward in an enterprise that started long ago, and which appears to have no end. My purpose from the beginning, and in all my work, has been to organize the disorderly material of our field so as to reveal the conceptual structure that gives it coherence and meaning. By the very nature of the task any success in performing even a part of it must be temporary, and any step forward only the beginning of an even more arduous exploration.

Allow me, first, to briefly look back. In *Aspects of Medical Care Administration* I dealt with a selection of concepts and methods that are fundamental to determining the need for health care, and to specifying the manner in which this need is to be filled. In a subsequent work, *Benefits in Medical Care Programs*, I examined the effects of prepayment, the criteria that may be used to evaluate them, and the means by which the expected effects can be influenced to serve the public purpose. And now I propose to deal with what may be the most central issue of all: the quality of the care which, in all our private and public programs, we are bent on providing. Thus, as I continue, I also start anew.

The subject of quality assessment and monitoring is, of course, not new to me. I have dealt with it in much of my previous work, always with a view to providing a framework within which the many complexities of the subject could be smoothed out and understood. This is also the purpose of my new work; but the task now is much more difficult than it was before. In recent years research in quality assessment has grown at an astounding pace, having attracted many investigators, among whom are some with considerable knowledge, inventiveness, and skill. We have also seen the implementation of large-scale public programs of quality assessment and monitoring, supplemented by many smaller programs that are privately run, and in which less traditional methods are often used. And all these activities have overwhelmed us with a flood of publications that are almost impossible to keep up with, let alone to assess as contributions to some larger design, especially since this muddy torrent of information seems to carry in its roiling rush an indiscriminate jumble of the new and the derivative, the meticulous and the careless, the honest and the manipulative, the well-informed and the unknowing, the wise and the perverse! Accordingly, the time seemed ripe for a review of the situation by one scholar who was familiar with the field, but who was also willing to begin with an open mind, and to take all the time that would be needed to separate the unsound from the wholesome, and to construct out of the latter a unified and inclusive structure.

In a moment of wild folly, which I have since bitterly regretted many times, I decided that I was that scholar. And, even more foolishly, I undertook the task hoping to complete it in a year or two, and to report my findings in one volume. But I soon found out that I had underestimated my assignment. For one thing, there was much more material to review than I had suspected. Then, this material was so uneven in quality and so varied in content that it took much longer to refine and organize it than I had expected. Moreover, as I should have anticipated, having had similar experiences in the past, the intellectual constructs that I brought to the task constantly failed me, so that, repeatedly, new frameworks for presenting and interpreting the material had to be developed. To me, this last experience was a source of reassurance and joy: reassurance that something new was being discovered, and joy in the act of discovery itself. But, all together, these several obstacles have slowed me down to a crawl. Therefore, I have had to revise drastically my schedule of work and my plans for publication. As to the former, I now realize that I must devote many more years to this enterprise; and I am reconciled to the prospect of perhaps not living long enough to complete it. As to the latter, it is clear that the result of my work must be published in parts. Each part, however, will cover a reasonably self-contained topic, and the successive parts will be published by the same publisher in a similar format, so that, gradually, a matching set of volumes will appear. And, needless to say, a strong thread of continuity will run through all these volumes, knitting them together into a whole.

This small volume is the first in the series that I have just described. It deals with the definitions of quality and the approaches to its assessment. It is, itself, divided into three parts.

The first part of this first volume is a conceptual exploration of the definition of quality itself. I began in this way because it seemed to me that at the very foundation of all our efforts to assess, to monitor, to protect, and to enhance the quality of care there ought to be a clear understanding of the nature of the thing itself on which all this attention was being so richly lavished. Somewhat to my surprise, what emerged is a model of quality that is capable of embracing in a unifying framework the two components of care, the technical and the interpersonal, as well as the content, the quantity, and the monetary cost of that care. This framework, especially when placed in a suitably defined context, can not only accommodate several equally valid views of quality, but it can also serve to identify and explain the similarities and differences among these views, and to point out their consequences to public policy. Finally, in this first part, I have attempted to explain, as a necessary basis for all subsequent discourse, my view of the relationship between quality assessment and program evaluation, of the manner in which accessibility, continuity, and coordination are included in, or excluded from, the definition of quality, and of the role that the satisfaction of clients and of practitioners plays in the definition of quality and in its assessment.

In the second part of this volume I enter the more concrete world of everyday experience in order to extract from the expressed opinions of clients, practitioners, and administrators, the views of quality which they share, as well as those on which they differ. Perhaps this "empirical" exploration is one way in which one can begin to translate the grand abstractions of the initial conceptual formulation into the more detailed attributes of care that represent its quality. What is more important, a commonality in views is necessary for a coherent approach to quality assessment and assurance; and where important disagreements are discovered, a way must be found to accommodate them in any scheme that one can hope will be seen as socially legitimate.

In the third part of this volume I attempt, yet one more time, to present the three approaches to quality assessment: structure, process, and outcome. But the emphasis now is not so much on describing these by now familiar approaches, as on testing their validity and usefulness. First, I attempt to show that a variety of alternative formulations of how quality may be assessed are fully congruent with the structure-process-outcome paradigm. Second, this paradigm is shown to have the capacity to organize and illuminate a number of rather detailed listings of the elements of care that have been proposed by other scholars as a means for assessing quality. Finally, I have carefully tested the two major contending approaches, process and outcome, by applying to each a set of criteria that I chose because they would reveal their similarities and differences, and because they would guide the choice of the more appropriate approach in any given situation. Happily, this systematic exploration of territory, that I thought was unlikely to hold any surprises for me, revealed new and unexpected treasures. Among these is the finding that process and outcome are fundamentally linked in a single, symmetrical structure that makes of one almost a mirror image of the other, no matter how many attributes are used to test the relationship. Thus, the emphasis shifts to a more thorough understanding of the linkages between process and outcome, and away from the rather misguided argument over which of the two is the superior approach to assessment.

The text of this first volume ends on this note. In the appendixes that follow I offer, based on my own earlier work, and on that of other scholars, a number of detailed listings of the elements of structure, process, and outcome that can be used to assess the quality of care. None of these listings, which are assembled for the reader's convenience, is intended to be a ready-made blueprint for assessment. My purpose is to provide a more detailed and concrete definition of the quality of care, and to guide the reader in devising the instrument that best meets his particular requirements.

This volume owes a great deal to the work of many friends and colleagues, whose contributions are carefully documented and whose influence is gratefully acknowledged. But my intent, in this volume and in the work that is to follow, is not merely to review the literature, but to make a personal statement that represents my own more mature thinking, and which I can leave behind as an affirmation of whatever it is that I stand for. I have, therefore, deliberately adopted a more than usually personal style. I have tried, more than I have in the past, to speak directly to the reader, hoping to establish a rapport that allows me to convey not only confirmed fact, but personal opinions and prejudices as well, provided each of these is honestly recognized for what it is. I would regret it deeply if, as a result of adopting this stance, I were seen by some to be unjustifiably opinionated or arrogant. On the contrary, what I want to reveal, hidden below the polished surface of his thought, is the scholar's vulnerable humanness: his hopes, his fears, and his doubts.

The best antidote to pride is a realization of one's indebtedness to others in the accomplishment of any task. This work is no exception. At the very beginning come the resources in money and time that must nourish the scholar. In that regard, I have been particularly fortunate. So far this work has been supported by the National Center for Health Services Research, under a grant that has undergone several modifications, as is indicated by the magical numbers 1-R01-HS-02081-01, 5-R01-HS-02081-02, 2-R01-HS-02081-03, and 3-R01-HS-02081-02S1. More recently, the Commonwealth Fund has generously agreed to join in supporting the preparation of the second volume in this series. As the work proceeds, the search for other sponsors must continue; and I will be deeply indebted to any who are able to help in this regard.

The University of Michigan has contributed to this volume through its regular grant of sabbatical leave, its willingness to make adjustments in my teaching and related responsibilities, and the availability of its superlative resources, among which the most important for this work has been the Reference Collection of literature in the organization of personal health services. As usual, Jack Tobias and Lillian Fagin have opened the rich treasures of the Reference Collection for my use, while Barbara Black has kept a steady and unerring hand on my finances.

The text of this volume owes a great deal to the sensitively meticulous editing of Margaret Thompson. She has tamed the grammatical and stylistic waywardness of my prose without muffling the distinctive voice with which I wanted to speak. Jean Thorby, with her usual skill and thoroughness, has verified all the references to the literature, and made of the indexes which she prepared a guide upon which the questing reader can assuredly depend. Everyone at the Health Administration Press has shown an openness to suggestions, a readiness to help, and a level of competence and good taste that have made the production of this book nothing less than a pleasure.

As I have already said, this monograph rests to a considerable extent on the original contributions of those scholars and researchers who are acknowledged in the text and in the lists of references. In preparing Chapter One, I had the opportunity to discuss my ideas with a good friend and colleague, Professor John Wheeler, and have benefited from his advice. This work probably also bears the imprint of still others, many of whom I can no longer identify, but who have influenced my thinking over the years. To all these I am deeply indebted. I must, however, accept full responsibility for what I have written, and absolve my sources and advisors of any contribution to the errors that I may have committed. In particular, this monograph does not in any way speak for the National Center for Health Services Research, or for The University of Michigan or any of its subunits. I hope, nevertheless, that it will not be found so wanting in merit that my friends and sponsors would want to utterly disown it!

And last, as well as first, I must acknowledge with deep gratitude the unfailing love and support of my wife and children, who have shared with me the burdens and privations of the scholar's vocation.

And now, a brief look forward. My next work, already about half completed, will be a study of the criteria which are the more specific representations of the concept of quality. Of course, this must be more than a simple description. It is necessary to find that set of the attributes of the criteria that will allow them to be classified and assessed. What I am looking for are the criteria of the criteria. And, if I am successful, something like a science of criteria may begin to take shape.

What lies farther in the dark future I cannot tell. I hope, however, that I shall be able to continue this work so that, in time, a great portion of the territory that comprises the field of quality assessment and monitoring will be suitably explored.

Meanwhile, as would any traveler just back from a fabled land, I want everyone to see what I have found. Will you, dear reader, give me your hand?

Come, let us go!

ONE

The Definition
of Quality: A
Conceptual Exploration

ONE

Introduction

To assess the quality of medical care one must first unravel a mystery: the meaning of quality itself. It remains to be seen whether this can be done by patiently teasing out its several strands or whether one must, in despair, use a sword to cut the Gordian knot.

Perhaps it is useful to begin with the obvious by saying that quality is a property that medical care can have in varying degrees. It follows that an assessment of quality is a judgment whether a specified instance of medical care has this property, and, if so, to what extent. What is by no means clear is whether quality is a single attribute, a class of functionally related attributes, or a heterogeneous assortment gathered into a bundle by established usage, administrative fiat, or personal preference. And the identity of the attribute or attributes that constitute quality is not clear at all. Moreover, even if the attributes can be identified, it would still be necessary to translate them into criteria and standards that can be used to make consistent judgments.

The definition and specification of attributes is, alas, only part of the problem. The phenomena or objects to which these attributes pertain are also poorly defined. There are different concepts of what constitutes "medical care" which, in their turn, lead to different formulations of what constitutes quality. Moreover, by extension, judgments of quality are often made not about medical care in itself, but indirectly about the persons who provide care, and about the settings or systems within which care is provided. As a result, the attributes of these persons and settings and the attributes of the care itself are used, alternately or simultaneously, both to define and to judge quality.

Given these ambiguities, it is no wonder that the quality of medical care has been perceived and defined in so many different ways. But these many variants are not a random assortment. There is an underlying conceptual structure that seems to embrace them all, revealing the sources of their similarities and the reasons for their differences. One purpose of this chapter is to construct and display that structure.

Basic Elements of a Definition

The search for a definition of quality can usefully begin with what is perhaps the simplest complete module of care: the management by a physician, or any other primary practitioner, of a clearly definable episode of illness in a given patient. It is possible to divide this management into two domains: the technical and the interpersonal. Technical care is the application of the science and technology of medicine, and of the other health sciences, to the management of a personal health problem. Its accompaniment is the management of the social and psychological interaction between client and practitioner. The first of these has been called the science of medicine and the second its art. But this terminology is not universally accepted, and it could be misleading. According to some, the technical management of illness can conjure up behaviors so mysteriously and elegantly appropriate as to me•it the appellation of "art." On the other hand, the management of the interpersonal relationship is an "art" mainly by default, because its scientific foundations are relatively weak, and because even the little that is scientifically known is seldom taught. Since technical care is neither completely nor exclusively a science and interpersonal care is capable of becoming at least in part a science, the distinction between science and art can be accepted only as an imperfect representation of the distinction between technical and interpersonal care.[1] The same can be said of the distinction between "care" and "cure," despite the alliterative euphoniousness of this terminology. Technical care is often far from curative; and it does not necessarily entail less caring than the management of the interpersonal process.

The terminology used is not, of course, as important as the general agreement on the usefulness of the distinction between the two domains of care. One should also note, however, that the two domains are interrelated, and that it may be difficult to make a distinction between them. It is easy to see how the interpersonal relationship can influence the nature and success of technical management. One could also plausibly suggest that the nature of the technical procedures used and the degree of their success will influence the interpersonal relationship. Finally, in the application of psychotherapeutic techniques the technical and interpersonal elements in management could be virtually inseparable. In most cases the distinction can be made, however, and is not only useful, but of fundamental importance to the definition of quality.

There may also be a third element in care which could be called its "amenities." This term could describe such features as a pleasant and restful waiting room, a comfortably warm examining room, clean sheets, a properly lubricated speculum that is neither too hot nor too cold, a comfortable bed, a telephone by the bedside, good food, and so on. It is not clear precisely how the category of the "amenities" is to be handled in a general model of quality. In a way, the amenities are properties of the more intimate aspects of the settings in which care is provided. But the amenities sometimes seem to be properties of the care itself. This becomes clearer when they are described in abstract form as comfort, promptness, privacy, courtesy, acceptability, and the like. In my own analysis the amenities will not receive separate attention, but will be considered primarily as part of, or contributions to, the management of the interpersonal relationship. This is because the amenities signify concern for patient satisfaction irrespective of whether they are provided directly by the practitioner, by the private practice which he controls, or by the larger organization of which the practitioner is an associate, a partner, or an employee.

So far, I have argued that quality is a property of, and a judgment upon, some definable unit of care, and that care is divisible into at least two parts: technical and interpersonal. It is necessary to say next what constitutes quality or goodness in each of these parts. At the very least, the quality of technical care consists in the application of medical science and technology in a manner that maximizes its benefits to health without correspondingly increasing its risks. The degree of quality is, therefore, the extent to which the care provided is expected to achieve the most favorable balance of risks and benefits.

What constitutes goodness in the interpersonal process is more difficult to summarize. The management of the interpersonal relationship must meet socially defined values and norms that govern the interaction of individuals in general and in particular situations. These norms are reinforced in part by the ethical dicta of health professions, and by the expectations and aspirations of individual patients. It follows that the degree of quality in the management of the interpersonal relationship is measured by the extent of conformity to these values, norms, expectations, and aspirations. But it could be argued that the consequence of this conformity is some form of social and personal good, and the absence of conformity a kind of loss. Moreover, to the extent that the interpersonal process contributes to the failure or success of technical care, it contributes to the balance of benefits and risks that flow from that care. Finally, a valuation of the benefits and risks, no matter what their nature, must be shared at least by the patient in addition to the practitioner responsible for the care. All these postulates lead us to a unifying concept of the quality of care as that kind of care which is expected to maximize an inclusive measure of patient welfare, after one has taken account of the balance of expected gains and losses that attend the process of care in all its parts. This concept is fundamental to the values, ethics, and traditions of the health professions: at the very least to do no harm; usually to do some good; and ideally to realize the greatest good that it is possible to achieve in any given situation.

How simple it all seems to be, and how reassuring to end our initial exploration in this way, at a pleasantly familiar resting place. But the simplicity and plausibility of this unifying concept of quality hides a great complexity beneath the surface. We must next look into these darker depths.

The Quantity of Care and Its Quality

One question that comes up early in a search for the meaning of quality is its relationship to the quantity of care. Obviously, access to care and the subsequent use of services must be taken into account when one is making judgments about quality. When care is received, but in amounts that are insufficient to bring about the realizable benefits in patient health and welfare, the care is clearly poor in quality because of quantitative inadequacy. When care is not received at all, though it should have been, there is going to be some difficulty with the analysis. There is obviously a failure of performance in some part of the system responsible for care, including the performance of the patient. But to put it this way is to accept a disturbing shift in the object of analysis, from the care itself to the system that provides it. The problem of passing a judgment on a non-existent episode of care can perhaps be solved in another way: by taking into account all the care received by a person over a longer period of time. In that case, a missing episode of care can easily fit in the category of insufficient care, denoting poor quality.

When care is said to be altogether unnecessary, or in some degree excessive, a judgment is being made that the care is not expected to make, as a whole or in some of its parts, a contribution to patient health or welfare. In addition to being useless, unnecessary care can also be harmful. Care that is both unnecessary and harmful is, of course, poor in quality, since the harm it is likely to cause is not balanced by any expectation of benefit. It is debatable whether there is, strictly speaking, such a thing as unnecessary but harmless care. But assuming that there is, should care that includes such a component be judged as poor in quality? There are several reasons for saying "Yes." First, such care is not expected to yield benefits. Second, it can be argued that it causes reductions in individual and social welfare through improper use of resources. By spending time and money on medical care the patient has less to use for other things he values. Similarly, by providing excessive care to some, society has less to offer to others who may need it more. Finally, the use of redundant care, even when it is harmless, indicates carelessness, poor judgment, or ignorance on the part of the practitioner who is responsible for care. It contra-- venes the rule of "parsimony," which has been, traditionally, the hallmark of virtuosity in clinical performance.[2]

We must therefore conclude that whenever a judgment is made about the necessity or suitability of the quantity of care a judgment of quality is implied. Assessments of the quantity and of the quality of care are thus inextricably intertwined, and will be so treated in this book.

Monetary Cost and the Quality of Care

The quality of care and its monetary cost are interrelated in several ways, among them the relationships between quantity and quality that I have described above. Obviously, quality costs money, since it presupposes quantitative adequacy and often means more care. When care is excessive and harmful, it is costlier but of poorer quality. When care is excessive, but the excess is harmless, it is costlier but without corresponding increases in quality, which makes for waste, as I have already remarked.

Care is also wasteful of resources, and costlier than it needs to be, when it is produced inefficiently. This happens, for example, when physicians do the work of nurses, or nurses the work of aides. It happens when a hospital is fully staffed but disproportionately occupied, or when it is either too small or too large to operate most efficiently. Thus, costs are increased, without corresponding increases in quality, because of inefficiencies in the methods and the scale of production.

It is clear from all this that monetary cost and quality are interrelated in a number of ways. To summarize, quality costs money, but it is possible by cutting out useless services and by producing services more efficiently to obtain higher quality for the money that is now spent on care, or to have the same quality at lower cost. We need not conclude, however, that monetary cost is an ingredient in the making of a judgment of quality itself. Monetary cost and quality do begin to overlap, in the conceptual sense, if one accepts the argument that unnecessary but harmless care, and care that is inefficiently produced, result in a loss in individual and social benefits because scarce resources are not put to their best use. But even here one could argue that inefficiency is to be distinguished from quality, even though its consequences affect the level of quality attained or attainable. A more persuasive case for monetary cost as an ingredient in the judgment of quality can be made if monetary cost is added to risk as an unwanted consequence of the provision of care. If we do this we will gain a more inclusive balancing of expected benefits and losses that can be used to define technical quality.

Benefits, Risk, and Cost: A Unifying Model

Figure 1-1 shows an attempt to pull together and develop several of these thoughts in a somewhat formal, though still hypothetical, model. In the upper panel of the Figure the volume of services is related to several variables. The first of these is benefits to health. The shape of the curve that relates the volume of services and benefits is, of course, unknown. I have assumed that as services are added there is, at first, a rapid increase in benefits and, later, a slowing down so that, toward the end, large additions to the services provided produce very small increases in benefits, or none. If benefits to health are used as the sole criterion of quality there is no clear-cut level of services which corresponds to optimum care. One must presumably continue to add services until no measurable additional benefits accrue. But that is to proceed without considering the risk that is inherent to a greater or lesser degree in all health care.

The hypothetical curve relating volume of services and risk to health, as shown in Figure 1-1, is roughly the mirror image of the path traced by benefits. The services prescribed and used first have large benefits and small risks. Then, as services are added, each increment has progressively larger risks and smaller benefits. If the postulates inherent in these curves are accepted, it is possible to plot for each additional step in the progression of services the health benefits minus the risks expected at that step — assuming, of course, that benefits and risks are measured in the same units. The result is shown in the lower panel of the Figure. The curve of "benefits minus risks" rises to a peak and then falls to zero, which is the point at which benefits equal risks. The most important feature of this curve is that it has a maximum point, which clearly identifies optimum quality. Of course, the shape of the benefit-minus-risk curve, and the position of its highest point, depend on the shapes of the curves of benefits and risks. These, in turn, are determined by the condition of the patient, the efficacy of medical science in respect to the care of that condition, and the degree of skill with which medical science is applied. Advances in medical science and technology, by definition, improve our ability to achieve greater benefits, lower risks, or both. When improperly or unskillfully applied, however, scientific innovations can also increase the potential to do harm without producing corresponding

FIGURE 1-1

Some Hypothetical Relationships Germane to the Definition of the Quality of Medical Care.

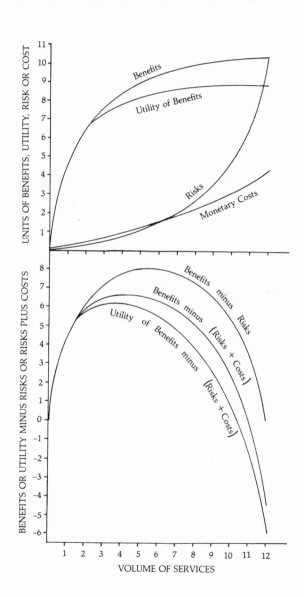

increases in benefits. But at any given state of medical science, the highest skill in its application is evidenced by the attainment of the highest possible benefits with the lowest possible risk at any given volume of service. This means that the curve of benefits minus risk will reach the highest possible peak; and the strategy of management that, on the average, achieves this result represents the highest level of quality, other things being equal. Anything less is less than perfect quality, but only convention and usage can fix the rough boundaries of what is meant when quality is judged to be "fair" or "poor." In the formulation illustrated by Figure 1-1 it is assumed that risks do not exceed benefits at any level of service, so that, at worst, health status is expected not to alter. In reality, risks can exceed benefits, so that there is a deterioration in health which is attributable to the care received. That this is poor quality no one would question.

It is important to emphasize that the peak in the curve of benefits minus risks represents the state of medical science as well as the way in which it is applied. This is important because the assessment of the efficacy of the science and technology must be carefully separated from the assessment of the quality of technical management. The latter is a judgment on how well the science and technology are used; quality, however, is not represented by health status, but by the extent to which the improvements in health status that are possible are realized.

It is now time to add to the analysis yet another variable: the cost of providing health services. The chart that appears in the upper panel of Figure 1-1 takes this variable into account.

Assume that it is possible to put a money value on the expected benefits and risks to health that correspond to any level of health services consumed. When this is done, it is possible to plot a curve that shows, at each level of services, the expected monetary value of benefits minus the sum of risks and monetary costs. The lower panel of Figure 1-1 shows this curve and how it compares to the curve of benefits minus risks. The new curve is shifted to the left, it extends below the zero line, and its peak is lower. In effect, a new standard has been established for the quality of technical management. This new standard has as a basis the postulate that monetary cost is an unwanted consequence of care and, for that reason, can be added to the expectation of risk in the assessment of the net benefit of technical management. The construction of the new standard also implies that monetary costs and benefits or risks to health are not incommensurate — that they can be valued in some comparable manner, even if only very roughly.[3]

Several of the factors that were mentioned earlier in the sections on quantity and quality and on monetary cost and quality will enter the model through their effect on benefits, risks, and monetary costs. The degree of efficiency in the production of services of course influences the relationship between cost and services that is pictured in Figure 1-1. Greater inefficiencies result in a steeper cost curve which, in its turn, produces a curve of benefits minus the sum of risks and costs which is shifted further to the left and has a lower peak. The use of unnecessary services will affect the curve in the same way, by lowering benefits and increasing risk relative to any level of monetary cost.

The final factor represented in Figure 1-1 is that of valuation or utility. It is postulated that individuals vary in the manner in which they value the expectations of health benefits, the risks, and the monetary costs that accompany the receipt of care in any condition. If this is so, there is another set of curves which represents these subjective valuations. For simplicity, I have shown only one of these in Figure 1-1: the valuation placed on the benefits. The consequence of using the value or utility of benefits rather than a more "objective" measure of benefits is shown in the lower panel of Figure 1-1. Under the assumptions implicit in the Figure, the shift of the net benefit curve is still further to the left and its peak is even lower. But these effects are to be taken only as an illustration of what could happen. What might actually occur depends on the relationship between benefits and the valuation of benefits. This relationship could be rectilinear, but is more likely to be curvilinear, so that the valuation of successive equal increments in health status becomes less and less. Actually, I assumed a relationship of this kind when I constructed Figure 1-1. Another important consideration is that the valuation of benefits, risks, and monetary costs might correspond in such a way as to leave their joint interrelationship unchanged. But this is unlikely. Patients and physicians are likely to vary in their propensity to incur risk in the expectation of a given benefit; and the valuation placed on monetary cost is likely to be more responsive than the valuation placed on increments of health status. But all this is hypothesis and therefore subject to empirical exploration.

The Unifying Model and Interpersonal Care

The unifying model was described as if it applied only to the quality of technical management. Nevertheless, as I have already pointed out, it is possible, at least hypothetically, to conceive of various strategies and styles in the management of the interpersonal process as having expected benefits and risks to one or several aspects of the patient's welfare. There are monetary costs as well, since the practitioner's personal attention requires time, and costly amenities must be added to assure comfort, privacy, convenience, and other things that contribute to the patient's satisfaction. It follows that curves similar to those shown in Figure 1-1 could be used to define a standard of the quality of interpersonal care. One argument for keeping this type of care separate as a measure of quality is the difficulty of expressing in a common unit of measurement the multiplicity of expected gains and losses in respect to the many objectives of care in the two forms of management. Important as this problem is, it is not a barrier to conceiving the possibility of one measure or standard of quality that is the final sum of all possible benefits, risks, and monetary costs that result from care. In fact, there is ample evidence in everyday experience that patients are able to assess the various benefits, risks, and costs within a common framework, and to make reasonable exchanges between one apparently nonmeasurable attribute and another. At the extreme, in acute, life-threatening illness, patients gladly relinquish many of the niceties of care, even though in retrospect they may resent deeply having had to do so. In certain chronic illnesses, where little improvement in physical function can be expected, and the main objective of care is to help the patient to cope with a disability, the elements that enter into the management of the interpersonal relationships become very important.

The Balance of Benefits and Risks in the Unifying Model

The balance of benefits and risks in the unifying model of quality is the result of several considerations. The first is the likelihood of occurrence of benefit or harm in any specified situation. The second is the magnitude of benefit or harm, which is the degree of deviation in health and welfare from what is expected in the absence of any health care intervention. Duration of benefit or harm can be seen either as a component of magnitude or as a separate entity. Promptness or delay in the occurrence of benefits or harm, together with duration, make up what might be called the time perspective on benefits and risks. This perspective is important because the valuations placed on benefits and risks can vary depending on whether these are immediate or delayed; and it is likely that individuals differ from each other in their relative preferences for the present as compared to the future. Clients and practitioners very probably take all of these factors into account, in a very rough and poorly understood way, in the decisions they make about what to do or not to do. But a more rigorous application of the model would require careful study and quantification of these factors.[4]

Some Implications of the Unifying Model

The unifying model asserts that individual expectations and valuations, as well as monetary cost, can enter the definition of the quality of care. I believe that these are indeed important considerations in the determination of what is the most appropriate care in actual practice. But, in addition to noting that these factors *can* and *do* enter the definition of quality, we need to consider whether they *should*. To define quality is to establish a norm; this means that the definition must be defensible on normative grounds.

Before adopting any position it would be useful to consider several alternatives. Of these, perhaps the simplest is to assert that health professionals should, as experts in the matter, have the prerogative of defining what is meant by "health status," what their intervention can contribute to health, and how that contribution is to be measured. The quality of medical care would then be defined as the management that is expected to achieve the best balance of health benefits and risks. It is the responsibility of the practitioner to recommend and carry out such care. All other factors, including monetary costs, as well as the patient's expectations and valuations, are thereby regarded as either obstacles or facilitators to the implementation of the standard of quality. They do not modify the standard itself. Though seldom explicitly expressed, this viewpoint is strongly represented when professional groups construct general formulations of the kind of care that constitutes quality. Nevertheless, I hesitate to call it the "professional" definition, because I do not believe it represents the full range of professional values and responsibilities. I do not want to call it the "technical" or "scientific" definition because I want to leave room for kinds of intervention or aspects of management that are not now considered to be scientific or technical. Perhaps it should be called the "absolutist" definition, since it has the fewest conditions attached to it.[5] It is conditional, however, on the nature of the health problem that is to be managed, and on the state of the science, technology, and "art" of medicine and its allied disciplines.

There is an alternative view. A long and honorable tradition of the health professions holds that the primary function of medical care is to advance the patient's welfare. If this is so, it is inevitable that the patient must share with the practitioner the responsibility for defining the objectives of care, and for placing a valuation on the benefits and risks that are expected as the results of alternative strategies of management. In fact, it can be argued that the practitioner merely provides expert information, while the task of valuation falls on the patient or on those who can, legitimately, act on his behalf. In principle, the patient, as the best judge of his own welfare, must direct the physician. In practice, the patient often will ask the health professional to act on his behalf. In that case the practitioner is expected not to substitute his own valuations for those of the patient, but to act in the best interests of the patient, considering what the practitioner knows or can find out about the patient's circumstances and valuations. Sometimes, the practitioner has good reason to believe that the patient is not in a position to make a proper assessment of the expected risks and benefits. For example, it may be impossible for the patient to predict how well he can adapt to an apparently crippling amputation, or to an operation that results in the loss of sexual function. Under these circumstances the practitioner should give the patient unbiased information about how other patients have responded to these disabilities and, if possible, arrange for the patient to meet with others who have had similar experiences. Since this is time consuming, the practitioner may be tempted to speed things up by "steering" the patient to a preconceived decision. But even such a decision must be, in the practitioner's opinion, the best, in the long run, for the patient. And in all these decisions, whether by the patient or on his behalf, the monetary cost of care and its impact on the patient's welfare is surely a legitimate and necessary consideration.

When the judgment of quality takes into account the patient's wishes, expectations, valuations, and means, we may speak of an "individualized" definition of quality, since patients differ considerably with respect to each of these. Patients are also different from one another in type and stage of illness, and in the demographic and social characteristics that influence the course of illness and its response to treatment. Given all these sources of variation, it is reasonable to ask whether it is possible to formulate specific, but generally applicable, criteria and standards of the quality of care. Many would argue that this is not possible, and would insist that the standard of quality must be established case by case.

One important consequence of using so many factors in the definition of the quality of care is the possibility that this will lessen the ability to formulate generalizable criteria and standards. The inclusion of monetary cost as a factor in this definition has other implications of its own. It is necessary to take cost into account whenever the patient pays at least a part of it, if the patient's net welfare is to be the criterion of quality. But including the monetary cost of care is tantamount to saying that the patient's ability to pay influences the standard of quality. This might be ethically acceptable if the benefits of care are enjoyed only by the patient, and if the distribution of incomes itself rests on an ethically justifiable foundation. If it is asserted that there is a right to medical care, even these justifications are insufficient. The inclusion of monetary costs as an ingredient in the "individualized" definition of quality, while necessary to that definition, does in consequence pose a moral problem for the practitioner, who must accept, in the interests of the patient, less than the greatest net benefit to health that medical science can confer. In fact, an analogous moral problem is created by any individual variation in the valuation of benefits and risks that is introduced because of social or economic factors whose distribution in the population could be considered inequitable. Thus the "absolutist" definition of quality is morally neutral, whereas the "individualistic" definition is not.[6] This may be why the formal pronouncements of medical leaders are couched in terms of the former, even though actual practice probably conforms more to the latter.

Of course, one can virtually remove monetary cost as a factor in the individualized definition of medical care by instituting some form of comprehensive health insurance, together with paid sick leave. The patient can in this case demand, and the practitioner provide, all the care that would make a net contribution to the patient's health and welfare. But the costs have not simply disappeared. They persist, important as ever, in the social sphere. And since society must, sooner or later, demand that costs be controlled, the practitioner, once again, faces a moral dilemma. On the one hand, there is his responsibility for, and commitment to, the patient's demand that he provide all the care that may do the patient good; and yet his responsibility to society, or his own dependence on social or institutional approval, demands that, because of monetary cost, he should stop somewhere short of the maximum health benefit attainable for any given individual.

This brings us to a third definition, which is the "social" definition of quality. The factors that produce this definition are the same as those that are used to get the "individualized" definition, but the quantities could be different. There is also a new criterion: in addition to the aggregate net benefit (or net utility) for an entire population, the social distribution of that benefit within the population becomes very important.

Differences between the "social" and the "individualized" definitions of quality arise in different ways. To the extent that monetary costs, for capital investment or for operations of a program, are shifted from individuals to the collectivity, or from one segment of the population to another, monetary cost would have a different impact on each of the two definitions. Another reason for the difference between the two definitions is that some forms of care are more highly valued at the social level than others because their benefits are felt by more people than just the individual who uses them. For example, elements of care that are introduced as part of planned research, formal education, or informal learning by trial and error might be held to be constituents of quality as socially defined, because they are expected to benefit others as well as the patient in the long run, even though they may not contribute to the immediate care of the patient. Finally, society may place different valuations on the health and welfare of different segments of the population distinguished by sex, occupation, and so on. This may reflect social values, economic considerations, or political influence and power. Social valuations, then, may rest on what is socially expedient rather than socially just. This raises still another ethical problem for the practitioner. It is one thing to ask the practitioner to place a limit on the care of some in the interest of fairness to all. It is quite another thing to require this in order to serve the interest of the economically privileged or the politically influential. There is a general presumption in democratic societies that social valuations represent a superior ethic. This may not always be the case.

Contextual Influences on the Definition of Quality

It is extraordinarily difficult to choose among the three definitions of quality: the "absolutist," the "individualized," and the "social." This may be because each definition is legitimate within an appropriate context. In fact, many differences in how quality is viewed and defined arise from differences in what might be called the scope and level of concern for the quality of care. Figure 1-2 is an attempt to illustrate this notion by showing some sources of the differences among the different perspectives, as well as showing certain similarities and interrelationships.

Figure 1-2 identifies three categories, each represented by one side of a cube: (1) the definition of health, (2) levels of aggregation and organization of the providers of care, and (3) levels of aggregation of the actual or potential recipients of care. Merely as an illustration, let us say that health is conceived to have three major components: physical-physiological function, psychological function, and social function. Also by way of illustration only, let us classify the providers of care as (a) a single practitioner, (b) several practitioners of the same or different professions or occupations, (c) a formally or informally organized team, or (d) an institution, plan, program, or entire system of medical care. As to the recipients, we will make two important distinctions: one between a "patient" and a "person," and another between the individual and the aggregate. A "patient" is a person who has actually received care during the period of time under review. A "person" is one who may or may not have received care during that period. The category of "person," therefore, includes that of patients, though the Figure, for simplicity, does not

FIGURE 1-2

SCHEMATIC REPRESENTATION OF A FRAMEWORK FOR
IDENTIFYING SCOPE AND LEVEL OF CONCERN AS
FACTORS IN DEFINING THE QUALITY OF MEDICAL CARE.

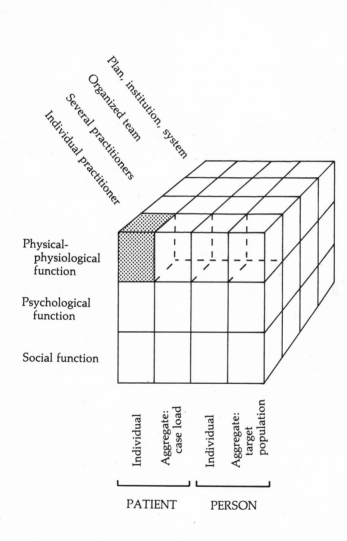

attempt to show this nesting of one category within the other. But, for each of these two categories, the Figure does show the further division into individuals and aggregates. A grouping of patients is called a "case load," while a group of persons is a target population, a community, or, even, a nation.

The implications of this formulation are reasonably direct. Traditionally, the object of concern in any definition or assessment of the quality of care has been the care provided by an individual practitioner, usually a physician, to an individual patient, with a view to improving or preserving physical-physiological function. This is represented in the Figure by the small, partially shaded cube at one corner of the larger construct. It is possible to enlarge one's scope of concern and, accordingly, to expand the definition of quality by espousing a broader concept of health that also includes aspects of psychological or social function. It is clear that the definition of quality and the definition of health will match one another, though not completely. They match only to the extent that the medical care system has been given, and has accepted, legitimate responsibility for human health and performance, together with the means to meet that responsibility. Aspects of "health" that are not within the purview of medical care are irrelevant to definitions or judgments of the quality of such care. At the extreme, "health" can be so broadly defined as to become synonymous with the "quality of life." In that case, judgments of the quality of medical care will pertain only to those legitimate medical care activities that contribute to the quality of life, and to no more; but also to no less.[7]

When several practitioners participate in the care of a patient, whether for a single episode or a succession, it may be necessary to assess the separate contribution of each provider. When the practitioners involved are from different professions and occupations, the definition of quality, and the methods used to assess it, must reflect the different roles, values, objectives, and technologies of the several participants. In addition, there should be greater attention given to the continuity and coordination of care. These attributes of the process of care are also relevant to care provided by one practitioner to a single patient, especially when there are several episodes of illness. But with several providers of care, failures in continuity and coordination are more likely; these attributes thereby become more important as determinants of the quality of care.

The distinction between patients and persons highlights the importance of access to care as a determinant of the quality of care when populations are the object of study. The distinction between individuals and aggregates emphasizes the importance of appropriate resource allocation as an attribute of the system that provides it. Access and resource allocation are, of course, interrelated, since differential access is one way in which resources are differentially allocated. But differences in consumption of resources can also arise after care has begun. The result, in either case, is that the quality of care is differentially distributed among individuals or segments of the population. This differential distribution is, obviously, an element of the "social" definition of quality, and a criterion for evaluating the performance of a program or system of health care. It is equally important as a criterion for evaluating the performance of each practitioner when his entire case load is the object of study. When one evaluates the performance of a practitioner case by case it is easy to slip into the assumption that his time, attention, and other resources are unlimited, and to expect that, in each case, the maximum attainable benefit is realized, including or excluding monetary cost as a factor. But when the entire case load is examined, the appropriate criterion of quality could be the net aggregate benefit. Thus, assessments of the performance of the individual practitioner in managing a case load, and of the performance of a program in serving a target population would become remarkably similar. Of course, it could be argued that neither the individual practitioner nor the program should take on more than can be managed at the highest level of quality for all. But, often, there is no real choice, since the alternatives are either near-perfect care for a few or less than perfect care for many.

It is clear that as the level and scope of concern move from the management of physical-physiological function by the individual to a progressively more inclusive framework, the concept of quality acquires successive envelopes of meaning. But some of these additions seem to be differences of emphasis rather than entirely new considerations. We have seen that the allocation of time and other resources affects the performance of individual practitioners as well as the performance of programs. The individual practitioner can also determine access to care by his location, his hours, and his charges, and by the way in which he deals with his patients and colleagues. These characteristics, in turn, influence the likelihood of his maintaining a stable and continuous relationship with his patient.

It is also debatable whether some of the considerations that come forward when the framework for analysis is expanded are really components of the definition of quality. For example, one could argue that continuity and coordination are desirable, not in themselves, but only if they contribute to the attainment of the highest net benefit or net utility. Similarly, access and resource allocation, important as they are, can be seen merely as instruments for use in the attainment of quality rather than as parts of the definition of quality itself.

I view these arguments with sympathy. There is the danger of enlarging the definition of quality so much that it loses distinctiveness and analytic utility, becoming almost a slogan which means nearly anything anyone chooses it to mean. Nevertheless, it is useful, at least for understanding why quality can mean so many different things to different people, to consider how changes in the level and scope of concern can alter one's perspective. Besides, certain important insights remain. It becomes perfectly evident that the manner in which health is defined, and the responsibility for health allocated, is of fundamental importance to a definition of what constitutes a relevant benefit or risk, and is therefore an ingredient in the definition of quality. It is also evident that the differences between the "individualistic" and the "social" definitions of quality remain, and that the two definitions are responses to different levels of responsibility and concern.

Quality Assessment and Program Evaluation

Differences in the definition of quality which result from differences in level and scope of concern are obviously pertinent to the relationship between quality assessment and program evaluation. If a program does not provide personal health services, the question of this relationship does not even come up, although evaluative activities of any kind have certain formal similarities — for example, they often involve the specification of a hierarchy of objectives, the determination of the degree to which objectives have been attained, and a consideration of how efficiently this latter has been done (Deniston et al. 1968a, 1968b). But we are not concerned with such purely formal analogies. Program evaluation and quality assessment are related in substance only when the program provides personal health services. If it does, it is important to consider whether the program has other functions as well. If the program also provides for professional education and health research, or for environmental health services as well, it is obvious that quality assessment pertains to only one of these functions, and that program evaluation must be much broader in scope. Quality assessment, under these circumstances, measures the success of the program in only one of its functions, the provision of personal health services.

When the program exists only to provide personal health services, one might expect program evaluation and quality assessment to be similar in extent. This is not necessarily so. Programs are implemented by organizations, and the assessment of organizational performance must account for activities related to organizational survival and growth, including financing, the recruitment of clients and employees, the maintenance of community acceptance and support, the cultivation of relationships with other agencies, and other adaptations to the organization's environment. Program evaluation must also account for the performance of the organizational subunits and their personnel whose function is to nourish, support, facilitate, and potentiate the activities of the units and personnel who provide health care directly to clients. What is even more important, the function of providing health services is viewed differently at the program level than it is at the level where clients and practitioners interact directly, irrespective of whether the program provides only health services or has other functions as well. Since most of these differences have already been discussed, only a summary is needed here.

What the differences are, and how large they are likely to be, depends on whether the program is designed to serve only patients (as in a hospital) or a population (as in a prepaid health plan, or a national health scheme). When responsibility is assumed for patients only, the definition of quality is not likely to differ in any fundamental way, but there is likely to be more attention given to access to care and to the allocation of resources. Certainly, efficiency in producing services, if it can be influenced by any factor that the organization can control, becomes very important. When the program serves a population, additional considerations will arise. The definition of quality is likely to be different because different valuations are placed on the benefits and risks of care. These differences are the consequence of an emphasis on the external benefits or disadvantages of care, and of a collective preference for a particular social distribution of the net benefits of care. Besides these considerations, there is likely to be concern for the social distribution of the costs of care. Equity, which is the assessment of who pays for as compared to who benefits from care, is an important element in the evaluation of certain programs, even though it does not figure in the definition of quality itself.

In most of the above measures, program evaluation appears to be more extensive, more inclusive, than quality assessment. This would not be true, however, with a program that provides only a small part of what is generally included in personal health services: for example, preventive services only, or health education only. In that case, the definition of quality, and the scope of assessment, is scaled down accordingly.

Having emphasized the differences between program evaluation and quality assessment, and between quality assessment at the program level and at the level of the client-practitioner interaction, I should also point out the similarities. Obviously, quality assessment is part of program evaluation — sometimes its most important part. The considerations that enter quality assessment at the level of the client-practitioner interaction become very similar to those at the program level if the practitioner is held responsible for the optimal management of his entire case load, or for a specified enrolled population. Furthermore, when quality assessment at the individual level reveals deficiencies in performance, the investigation of the reasons for these deficiencies will often lead outward and upward into the organization, involving many elements of program evaluation.

Accessibility, Continuity, and Coordination

In my discussion of the context of quality assessment I pointed out that as attention shifts from the interaction of one patient-practitioner pair to the provision of care by groups of practitioners to entire populations, a number of attributes of care become much more prominent determinants of the quality of care. Among these I mentioned accessibility, continuity, and coordination. It is now time to consider what these attributes are, and how precisely they are related to the definition of quality.

Care may be said to be accessible when it is easy to initiate and to maintain. Of course, accessibility depends on the properties of the providers of care — whether these are institutions or individuals — that make them more or less easy to get to and use. But it also depends on the ability of potential clients to overcome the financial, spatial, social, and psychological obstacles that intervene between clients and the receipt of care. Accessibility thus involves an adaptation between the providers and the clients of care which facilitates their conjunction.[8] And this, in turn, influences the quality of care in ways that have already been discussed. Briefly, quality is influenced through the quantity of services and the types of services recommended by the practitioners and accepted by the patient. Quality is also influenced through the social distribution of services and their benefits. The cost of care, to the extent that it is borne by the patient, is a factor that influences accessibility, and is also a part of the definition of quality, as I have shown. In all these ways, accessibility and quality are closely related. But this is not to say that they are the same thing. I believe that it is more appropriate to separate the two phenomena, defining the accessibility of care as the ease with which it is initiated and maintained, and defining the quality of care as its expected ability to achieve the highest possible net benefit according to the valuations of individuals and of society. With this separation, each concept is more specific and, I believe, more useful as a tool in analysis. For example, although greater accessibility is usually associated with greater quality, it could also lead to redundant, harmful, or unnecessarily costly care. Furthermore, greater accessibility of care to some segments of the population could mean either greater or lower quality depending on the criteria that govern the social valuation of the distribution of health benefits.

I am inclined to view the relationship between quality and continuity or coordination in much the same way as I view the relationship between quality and accessibility. Coordination may be regarded as the process by which the elements and relationships of medical care during any one sequence of care are fitted together in an overall design. Continuity means lack of interruption in needed care, and the maintenance of the relatedness between successive sequences of medical care (Shortell 1976; Bass and Windle 1972). A fundamental feature of continuity is the preservation of information about past findings, evaluations, and decisions, and the use of these in current management in a way that indicates stability in the objectives and methods of management, or their orderly and reasonable evolution.[9] Coordination involves the sharing of such information among a number of providers to achieve a coherent scheme of management. It is believed that continuity and coordination are better if responsibility is centralized, as much as possible, in the hands of one practitioner and, when more than one practitioner or source of care are involved, if a legitimate and orderly apportionment or transfer of responsibility is arranged. It is also believed that coordination and continuity of care lead to a better understanding of the patient's medical care problem, his situation in general, and his values and expectations. All this results in more appropriate clinical decisions, and a greater likelihood that the patient will participate effectively in care, and be satisfied with it. To the extent that duplication is avoided, costs will also be reduced. All of these consequences, if present, would improve the quality of care, defined in terms of expected net benefit as valued by the patient.

But, at least hypothetically, it is also possible that continuity will result in lack of attention to new developments in the patient's situation, a persistence in past omissions and errors, and the perpetuation of a less than fully desirable client-practitioner relationship. From these considerations, I draw the conclusion that quality can be defined independently of coordination and continuity. However, it could be that coordination and continuity cannot be defined independently of quality. If continuity means noninterruption of needed care, the decision that care is needed involves a judgment of quality. Similarly, the search for consistency, orderly evolution, or design in the sequence of care and in its contemporaneous patterning seems difficult without some concept of "rational" care, which is, itself, a representation of quality. This suggests that, at least in some ways, the concept of quality cannot be fully separated from the more fundamental formulations of continuity and coordination.[10] This is not true, of course, when continuity and coordination are defined more simply (and superficially) as the use of one source of care, or as an orderly transfer from one source to another. Continuity and coordination of responsibility for care are clearly separable, as concepts, from the definition of quality, even though the former two could be important determinants of the achievement of good performance. It is also conceivable that, in some cases, a fundamental initial mistake determines the entire course of subsequent care, which remains continuously and consistently confirmed in error. This would be a kind of logical continuity that is, nevertheless, wedded to poor quality. One hopes that this kind of continuity, though conceptually of great interest, is very unusual in practice.

Let me recapitulate: I would like to take the position that accessibility, continuity, and coordination are attributes of care that influence its quality but remain separate from it. I am not prepared to argue that this is the only correct or reasonable formulation. A case could be made for including accessibility, coordination, and continuity as integral parts of the definition of quality. I prefer to keep the several concepts distinct and separate partly because I need to scale down the scope of this work to something less unmanageable than it already is. I also believe that maintaining the distinctions will be helpful in subsequent analysis and discussion.

Clients and the Definition of Quality

Obviously, clients individually and collectively contribute in many ways to the definition of quality. One way is by influencing what is included in the definitions of "health" and "health care." It is generally believed that clients tend to have a broader view of these things and, as a result, they expect more from the practitioner than the practitioner is willing or able to give. Sometimes the client may have a narrower view. He will then resent and resist what he will consider an intrusion into private matters that should not be the practitioner's concern. Clients also contribute to the definition of quality, as the unified model shows, by determining the valuations that are to be placed on the expected benefits and risks to health. They do this as individuals, if the individualistic definition of quality is adopted, and as a collectivity in the social definition of quality. Of course, clients also contribute very heavily to the definition of quality with their values and expectations regarding the management of the interpersonal process. In this domain, clients, individually and collectively, are the primary definers of what quality means.

In recognition of all these considerations, client satisfaction is often seen as an important component of the quality of care. In this regard, it is a curiously complex phenomenon. In one sense, client satisfaction or dissatisfaction correspond to the healing of a wound or the mending of a bone. Each function defines a state of the patient which is a consequence rather than an attribute of care. As such, satisfaction can be seen as an element of psychological health; this makes the achievement of the maximum attainable satisfaction one objective of care.

Client satisfaction, besides being an objective and outcome of care in its own right, can also be seen as a contribution to other objectives and outcomes. For example, a satisfied client is more likely to cooperate effectively with the practitioner, and to accept and adhere to his recommendations. Satisfaction also influences access, since the satisfied client is thought to be more likely to seek care again.

Client satisfaction has still another role in quality assessment. It can be regarded as the patient's judgment on the quality or the "goodness" of care. It represents the client's assessment of quality in a way that corresponds to a professional's assessment of the quality of the same care, even though the considerations that enter the two judgments may not be the same, and the conclusions may differ. The client's assessment of quality, expressed as satisfaction or dissatisfaction, could be remarkably detailed. It could pertain to the settings and amenities of care, to aspects of technical management, to features of interpersonal care, and to the physiological, physical, psychological, or social consequences of care. A subjective summing up and balancing of these detailed judgments would represent overall satisfaction.

Client satisfaction is of fundamental importance as a measure of the quality of care because it gives information on the provider's success at meeting those client values and expectations which are matters on which the client is the ultimate authority. The measurement of satisfaction is, therefore, an important tool for research, administration, and planning. The informal assessment of satisfaction has an even more important role in the course of each practitioner-client interaction, since it can be used continuously by the practitioner to monitor and guide that interaction and, at the end, to obtain a judgment on how successful the interaction has been. But client satisfaction also has some limitations as a measure of quality. Clients generally have only a very incomplete understanding of the science and technology of care, so that their judgments concerning these aspects of care can be faulty. Moreover, clients sometimes expect and demand things that it would be wrong for the practitioner to provide because they are professionally or socially forbidden, or because they are not in the client's best interest. Even these limitations do not necessarily rob patient satisfaction of its validity as a measure of quality, though.

For example, if the patient is dissatisfied because his unreasonably high expectations of the efficacy of medical science have not been met, one could argue that the practitioner has failed to educate the patient. And when the patient is dissatisfied because a desired service has been denied, the grounds for that denial could be of questionable validity, especially if it is assumed that the primary responsibility of the practitioner is to the individual client, and that the client is, ultimately, the best judge of his own interests, provided he is mentally unimpaired and properly informed.

These considerations, taken together, show that client satisfaction is related to quality in a number of ways. To the extent that client satisfaction is a distinct benefit of care, it figures in the balance of benefits and harms that is the fundamental core of the definition of quality. To the extent that client satisfaction contributes to other benefits because it influences access or adherence to the regimen of care, it occupies a secondary position in the definition of quality, since the benefits to which it contributes can be measured more directly. To the extent that client satisfaction is a judgment on the quality of care, it is not part of the definition of quality. It is, however, the best representation of certain components of the definition of quality, namely, those which pertain to client expectations and valuations.

Practitioner Satisfaction

To maintain symmetry, if for no other reason, we must consider how the degree of satisfaction of the practitioners is related to the definition of quality. A sense of general satisfaction may be conducive to the best performance of the practitioner. Practitioner satisfaction, like client satisfaction, is also, partly, a judgment of "goodness" that pertains to the settings and conditions of the practitioner's work, to the care provided by colleagues, and to the care given by the practitioner himself, in general or in any particular instance. Practitioner satisfaction, then, is either a causal factor of good care or a judgment on the goodness of care. In neither capacity is it a component of the definition of "goodness" itself.

The definition of quality, as presented in this chapter, rests solely on the extent to which the client's interests have been advanced. Nevertheless, the organization as whole, if it is to survive and grow, must also serve the interests of practitioners. In this context, practitioner satisfaction becomes a criterion of the quality of certain features and functions of the organization (Freeborn and Greenlick 1973).

Choosing a Definition of Quality

The analysis I have made up to this point leads to the conclusion that there are several definitions of quality, or several variants of a single definition; and that each definition or variant is legitimate in its appropriate context. While this formulation is useful for analysis, it does not help as a guide to public policy or personal action. For example, there is still the question of which definition should be espoused by a health professional who provides personal health services for which he is responsible, and by the professional association that legitimizes the practitioner's point of view. I feel that, having raised the issue, I am obligated to express an opinion, even it if is tentative.

I am convinced that the balance of health benefits and harm is the essential core of a definition of quality. I am reasonably certain that harm and benefits must be compared primarily as they are valued by the fully informed patient or his legitimate representative. A good case can also be made for using the avoidance of useless care (which, incidentally, also lowers cost) as an element of the definition of quality. The efficiency of production, to the extent that it is determined by factors other than practitioner decisions in the management of individual patients, should be excluded from the definition of quality, though it remains an important consideration in its own right. As to the social valuations placed on health benefits and risks, I believe that these should be excluded if they differ from individual valuations, in order to avoid diluting the loyalty of the practitioner to the individual patient. Social valuations that differ from individual valuations should be expressed by resource allocation at the aggregate level, including the institution of special programs, special benefits, and the like. The responsibility of the practitioner would then be to do his best for each patient, within the framework of social constraints and facilitations.

The only element in the definition of quality that remains truly problematic is the role of monetary costs as balanced against net benefits to health. I believe that, in real life, we do not have the option of excluding monetary costs from the individualized definition of quality. Their inclusion means that the practitioner does for each patient what the patient has decided his circumstances allow. In so doing, the practitioner has discharged his responsibility to the patient, provided that he has helped the patient to discover and use every available means of paying for care. It is true that this may result in a distribution of care and the benefits of care that is inequitable, or less than socially optimal. But this problem can be solved only by social action. When this action entails the imposition of controls over the use of health services, it is the practitioner's role, as I see it, to act as the patient's advocate, so that the system can be made most responsive to each patient's interests. The consequence is an inevitable tension between the practitioner and the mechanisms of social control, which implies conflict between the individualized and the social definitions of quality.

It seems to me that this conflict between the individualized and the social definitions of quality can be resolved if the direct and indirect costs of care are borne by society, and if, at the same time, the practitioner is made responsible for the welfare of an entire group of people. We could then apply an ethically defensible social definition of quality. According to this definition, all person-years of life at full function would be equal in value.[11] All persons would have equal access to care, but would contribute to the costs of care in a manner that is equitably related to their ability to pay. Given a specified quantity of resources devoted to medical care, the highest quality of care would be that which yields the highest net utility for the entire population. It is the responsibility of the professional schools to discover and to teach those strategies of care that are most likely to achieve this result. When this happens, the care provided to each individual, in accordance with these strategies, would conform to the social standard of quality.

I am not sure that this Utopian solution is fully realizable. Until it is implemented, it seems inevitable that the individual practitioner will be subject to the conflict engendered by the simultaneous application of the three definitions of quality: the absolutist, the individualized, and the social.

Notes to Chapter One

[1] The alternative view is well represented by Brook and Williams, who define quality of care as follows:

$$\begin{pmatrix} \text{"Quality} \\ \text{of} \\ \text{Health} \\ \text{Care} \end{pmatrix} = \begin{pmatrix} \text{Technical} \\ \text{Care} \end{pmatrix} + \begin{pmatrix} \text{Art} \\ \text{of} \\ \text{Care} \end{pmatrix} + \begin{pmatrix} \text{Technical} \\ \text{Care} \end{pmatrix}\begin{pmatrix} \text{Art} \\ \text{of} \\ \text{Care} \end{pmatrix} + \epsilon$$

Here, technical care includes the adequacy of the diagnostic and therapeutic processes. Art-of-care relates to the milieu, manner, and behavior of the provider in delivering care to and communicating with the patient. The interactive term emphasizes the notion that the two terms are not just additive. Finally, an error term is included as a reminder that a measurement of any construct, such as quality, includes random error...." (Brook and Williams 1975, p.134)

² In a manuscript on quality assurance of health services that is being prepared for the European Office of the World Health Organization, Vuori elevates this notion to a separate category of "logical quality." According to him, "The concept of logical quality...is derived from information theory and refers to the efficiency with which information is being used in arriving at a decision. The less information is needed to establish a diagnosis, the better is the logical quality....From the point of view of information theory, too much information and irrelevant information is not only costly but may also turn out to be dysfunctional by constituting 'noise' that may hamper the proper utilization and interpretation of the necessary information. The concept of logical quality can also be applied when analyzing the utilization of manpower....The use of over-competent personnel certainly lowers the logical quality of the activities and increases their costs." (Page 43 of manuscript) My own appreciation of the principle of parsimony derives not from information theory, of which I am innocent, but from the precepts and example of my clinical teachers, and from a no more than nodding acquaintance with William of Ockham, who used the Law of Parsimony (which we know as Occam's razor) to justify a ruthless paring away of all that he considered to be superfluous in explaining reality.

³ It seems that in recent years several scholars have arrived at essentially similar formulations of the role of monetary cost in the definition of quality. One example is to be found in the work of Vuori cited in the preceding Note. (See pages 37–43 of Vuori's manuscript.) In addition to considering the consequences of including or excluding costs in the definition of quality, Vuori raises the question of whether optimal quality is the level of services that maximizes net benefit minus cost or the level that maximizes the ratio of net benefits to cost. He finds it obvious that the consumer would prefer the first, while the "producers" would prefer the second. Another similar formulation has been advanced by Havighurst and Blumstein, who emphasize the differences in health policy that result not only from including monetary costs in the definition of quality, but also from distinguishing private costs from social costs (Havighurst and Blumstein 1975, pp.15–20).

⁴ An excellent example of this kind of empirical study is a paper by McNeil et al. (1978) that shows how the valuation placed by patients on immediate risk, relative to future advantages, influences the preference for surgery to radiation therapy in the management of lung cancer.

⁵ In the work cited in Notes 2 and 3, Vuori also uses the term "absolute quality" to describe the standard of quality when "we omit...the significance of the economic factors to the parties concerned." (Page 39 of manuscript)

⁶ It seems to me that the "absolutist" definition is morally neutral only in the sense that it is a technical solution to a technical problem. Yet the assertion that the optimal solution must be found and applied represents a moral stance which is not perceived to involve moral choice only because it is such a universal and unquestioned norm of the medical profession.

⁷ Brook comments on this subject as follows: "The phrase, quality of care, is vague and has acquired various emotional overlays. Some people use these words

to be synonymous with quality of life. This means that ideals such as liberty, happiness, and individual autonomy become components of quality of care; consequently, any valid measurement of quality must take into account these different ideals. . . . For purposes of this paper, only measures of that component of health which can be altered by the medical care system will be considered as indicators of quality of care. Quality of care, then, differs from quality of life." (Brook 1973, pp.114-15) I believe that Brook and I agree that the quality of care is not coextensive with the quality of life. It is possible, however, that I am placing a little more emphasis on the need to include those aspects of the quality of life to which medical care can make a contribution. Moreover, some attributes that are part of the quality of life — for example, the maintenance of autonomy and self-respect — are also attributes of a desirable client-practitioner relationship and, in this way, become part of the definition of quality.

[8] For a more detailed discussion of this formulation as it applies to socioorganizational and geographic accessibility see Donabedian 1973, pp.419-56.

[9] For studies of continuity and coordination that use as a criterion the preservation, recognition, and use of past information see Starfield et al. 1976 and 1977, and Simborg et al. 1976.

[10] I believe that Bass and Windle as well as Shortell run into this kind of difficulty. For example, Bass and Windle say, "We have defined continuity of care as the relatedness between past and present care in conformity with the therapeutic needs of the client." (Bass and Windle 1972, p.111) According to Shortell, "Continuity of medical care can be defined as the extent to which medical care services are received as a coordinated and uninterrupted succession of events consistent with the medical care needs of the patients." (Shortell 1976, p.378) Both of these definitions give a central position to the adaptation of care to the needs of the patient. But when this is done, continuity becomes, *by definition*, always good and, therefore, necessarily linked to quality. In order to break this tie one must be able to conceive of "a coordinated and uninterrupted succession of events" which show "relatedness between past and present care" without *necessarily* being *appropriately* related to the needs of the patient. The only way this can be done is to admit the possibility of uninterrupted care that follows an internally consistent but erroneous course of management.

[11] The meaning and implications of this assumption are discussed and illustrated in Donabedian (1973), pages 136-192.

References to Chapter One

Bass, R.D., and Windle, C., "Continuity of Care: An Approach to Measurement." *American Journal of Psychiatry* 129 (1972):110-15.
Brook, R.H., "Critical Issues in the Assessment of Quality of Care and Their Relationship to HMOs." *Journal of Medical Education* 48 (1973):114-34.
————, and Williams, K.N., "Quality of Health Care for the Disadvantaged." *Journal of Community Health* 1 (1975):132-56.

Deniston, O.L.; Rosenstock, I.M.; and Getting, V.A.; "Evaluation of Program Effectiveness." *Public Health Reports* 83 (1968):323–35. [1968a in text]
———; Rosenstock, I.M.; Welch, W.; and Getting, V.A.; "Evaluation of Program Efficiency." *Public Health Reports* 83 (1968):603–10. [1968b in text]
Donabedian, A., *Aspects of Medical Care Administration: Specifying Requirements for Health Care.* Cambridge, Mass.: Harvard University Press, for the Commonwealth Fund, 1973. 649 pp.
Freeborn, D.K., and Greenlick, M.R., "Evaluation of the Performance of Ambulatory Care Systems: Research Requirements and Opportunities." *Supplement to Medical Care* 11 (1973):68–75.
Havighurst, C.C., and Blumstein, J.F., "Coping with Quality/Cost Trade-Offs in Medical Care: The Role of PSROs." *Northwestern University Law Review* 70 (1975):6–68.
McNeil, B.J.; Weichselbaum, R.; and Pauker, S.G.; "Fallacy of the Five-Year Survival in Lung Cancer." *New England Journal of Medicine* 299 (1978):1397–1401.
Shortell, S.M., "Continuity of Medical Care: Conceptualization and Measurement." *Medical Care* 14 (1976):377–91.
Simborg, D.W.; Starfield, B.H.; Horn, S.D.; and Yourtee, S.A.; "Information Factors Affecting Problem Follow-Up in Ambulatory Care." *Medical Care* 14 (1976):848–56.
Starfield, B.H.; Simborg, D.W.; Horn, S.D.; and Yourtee, S.A.; "Continuity and Coordination in Primary Care: Their Achievement and Utility." *Medical Care* 14 (1976):625–36.
———; Simborg, D.; Johns, C.; and Horn, S.; "Coordination of Care and Its Relationship to Continuity and Medical Records." *Medical Care* 15 (1977):929–38.
Vuori, H., "Quality Assurance of Health Services." Unpublished manuscript, March 23, 1978. (To be published by the World Health Organization, Regional Office for Europe, Copenhagen.)

TWO

The Definition
of Quality: Some
Empirical Studies

TWO

There is an overabundance of more or less fanciful opinions, among them my own, about what quality means or what it should mean. I wish there were as much attention given to studying how clients, practitioners, administrators, and policy makers define quality when asked to do so, and what definitions can be inferred from their actual behavior. All of these definitions, as well as the differences and similarities among them, are bound to be important factors in the organization, provision, and use of health care services. But this subject has not been altogether neglected; and while there is little work that deals with it directly, there is a great deal that touches on it. In this chapter I shall review only a selection of studies that touch on the subject, and in each study I will deal only with those aspects that bear on the definition of quality. I am unable to do more now. It seems to me, nevertheless, that it would have been useful to review more thoroughly the extensive literature that deals with the opinions of clients and providers, with the express purpose of inferring how they define quality.

The Clients' View of Quality

People are seldom asked to say what they think the quality of medical care means. The question is put indirectly. What is a good doctor, nurse, or clinic? What is a bad one? What does the respondent like and dislike about his doctor, nurse, clinic, and so on? From these opinions about the attributes of providers inferences must be drawn about the ingredients of "goodness" in the care they give. In order to make the task simpler, the respondent is often given a list of attributes and asked to rank all these or to select some. When this is done, the questioner's view of the boundaries and content of the concept of quality may be imposed on the respondent.

Moreover, the respondent's answers are influenced by his interpretation of the language in which the choices are presented. Finally, studies of this kind often deal with particular populations in special situations. When this is the case, it is not clear how generally applicable the findings are.

Much of the literature on client views of the good doctor or clinic pertains to the relative importance of the technical management of illness as compared to the management of the relationship between the client and the practitioner. In the early 1950s, Rose Laub Coser, a sociologist, put on the white robe that signifies clinical authority and became what she thought was a "neutral" observer in the medical and surgical wards of "Mount Hermon," a hospital in a metropolitan area in the eastern United States. In addition, she conducted "standardized interviews" with 51 patients at discharge. The result is a fascinating account of how patients adapt to the hospital, and what they think of their doctors and nurses (Coser 1956, 1962).

When Coser asked "What is your idea of a good doctor?" the answers given by the patients seemed to classify them into two rather distinct groups. A little more than half the patients saw the good doctor as one who provided kindness, love, and security. He "talks nice," takes an interest, makes you "feel good," or is so all-knowing and all-powerful that you can rest secure in his safe-keeping. By contrast, a little less than half dwelled on the doctor's "scientific and professional competence." The patients appeared similarly divided in their view of the hospital. Some saw it as a place meant and equipped to do the job of treating illness better than it could be done outside the hospital. Others thought of it as a place where they received care and attention, "a home away from home," which they enjoyed and were sometimes reluctant to leave. A twofold division also emerged in answer to the question, "What makes a good patient?" A little over half seemed to think that the good patient should be to some degree autonomous, whereas almost all the rest seemed to think that the patient should be completely submissive. And most significantly, in Coser's view, these several dichotomies did not divide the patients haphazardly, but were interrelated, so that it was possible to show an overall division into two types of persons. There were those who thought the hospital had the rather limited technical task of caring for illness, who also defined the doctor's goodness in technical-professional terms, and saw the patient as rather autonomous, as well. And there were the others, who saw the hospital as another, sometimes better, home, who defined the doctor's goodness in terms of kindness, personal interest, and care, and who saw the patient's own role as one of unquestioning acceptance.

Coser's work shows remarkable sensitivity and insight, but one can question the general applicability of her conclusions. It is possible that her findings reflect the particular characteristics of her subjects, whom she describes as generally elderly, poor, Eastern European Jews, who were strangers in "their" hospital, separated by a social chasm from their doctors, and also estranged from the rapidly changing ways of life of those around them in the outside world.

Partial support for Coser's dichotomies may be inferred from a study made at the Hadassah Hospital in Jerusalem (Shiloh 1965). When asked to say what was happening in each of four sketches that depicted common hospital situations, patients replied in a manner that led Shiloh to distinguish two kinds of patients whom he called "equalitarian" and "hierarchal." Those who were in the first category saw themselves as equal partners with the hospital, expecting to be informed about their condition and to participate in making decisions. They were satisfied with the technical aspects of care, but critical of the "impersonal, non-communicative" way in which it was conducted, and resentful of their own passivity as recipients. They complained about the hospital environment, including its noisiness, its lack of cleanliness, and the unpalatability of the food; and they looked forward to going home. By contrast, those in the second category, whom Shiloh called "hierarchal," thought of themselves as passive, grateful recipients of care. They were impressed by the technical apparatus of the hospital, and were so pleased with its amenities and comforts that they were in no hurry to leave, sometimes being afraid of early discharge. Besides, many had personal problems, familial or financial, which they expected the hospital to help them solve.

The division of patients into two types and the adjustment of the practitioner's style of management to the preferences of each (or the assignment of each type of patient to a corresponding type of practitioner) would, of course, be a very important element in the individualized definition of quality, as presented in the opening chapter of this monograph. Unfortunately, other researchers have not looked for this differentiation into types or, having looked, have failed to find it. Among the latter is Freidson's classic study of the members of a hospital-based prepaid group practice in The Bronx, New York (Freidson 1961). The enrollees represented a wide range of educational and occupational positions, from professors and professionals to semiskilled workers with grade school education. Half of them were Jewish and the rest Catholic and Protestant, in that order, with large Italian and Irish minorities. Traditionally middle class in background and orientation, these people were suspicious of strangers and fearful of being pushed around. They valued independence, thrift, and an almost obsessive cleanliness. They were concerned about health and were prone to become agitated or frightened at the prospect of even minor illness, especially in children. In many of these characteristics, the people studied by Freidson seem not unlike a large

majority of the U.S. population, but the fact that the former were enrolled in a prepaid group practice plan does make the setting, if not the
people, somewhat atypical.

In this setting, Freidson was able to force a choice on a representative
sample of enrollees to whom he administered a formal questionnaire. "If
you had to pick one doctor out of a group, what kind would you choose?"
he asked. In reply, some chose the alternative which said, "The smartest
and best doctor, and I wouldn't care too much whether he took personal
interest in me or not." Others selected "the best personality, the one
who'd take the most personal interest in me." Unfortunately, we are not
told what proportion of respondents chose each of the two alternatives;
but we do know that only 15 percent rejected both alternatives, selecting
instead a third one which said, "Other," and which invited the respondent to give an explanation.[1] However, the willingness to settle for the
"smartest and best" or "the one who'd take the most personal interest,"
does not necessarily mean that there are two types of patients with fundamentally different views of the quality of care. This is particularly so
in a situation where the organization has already paid a great deal of attention to the recruitment of "good physicians." At best, the responses
might indicate a preference for an extra bit of competence as compared to
an extra amount of personal interest. Freidson's own conclusion, based
on intensive interviews with 36 families, and many months of observation of patients and physicians, was that, in reality, people wanted both
"personal interest" and "competence." And while the two attributes, personal interest and competence, were distinguishable properties, and
could be discussed separately, patients insisted that one could not exist
without the other. In a sense, personal interest provided the assurance
that the doctor's competence was being fully used in the interests of the
patient. Obviously, this is an interpretation that fits well with the unifying model of quality as described in Chapter One. And further exploration of what people include under the headings of personal interest and
competence shows that clients, as expected, subscribe to highly individualized definitions of the quality of care.[2]

Freidson's reconstruction of what patients want and value in their doctors and in the care they provide emerged mainly from lengthy interviews in which people spoke freely about their experiences in receiving
care in the prepaid plan and outside it, including their reasons for liking
or disliking certain doctors, and for continuing to receive care from one
but not from another.[3] To the patient, "personal interest" means that the
doctor treats him as a person having his own identity, and respects him
as such, showing care and concern in handling his individual problems in
an individualized manner. Some patients appreciate "a joking familiar-

ity," and others a respectful reserve, but all object to mechanical, routinized, impersonal handling. There is evidence of personal interest when the physician takes time, and is deliberate and careful. People dislike the physician who is "curt" or "abrupt," who treats the patient in a "cursory way," or rushes him in and out. Communication is important as a condition of personal interest. The doctor must be willing, and take time, to hear and answer questions, and to explain. Equality of status is still another condition. The patient expects to be treated with courtesy and respect, and as a person capable of making intelligent choices, provided the physician explains the alternatives.

According to Freidson, "patients assume that all doctors possess a minimal competence," and they are concerned only with degrees of competence. Patients seem even more interested in the full exercise of existing competence on their behalf. The problem seems to be not so much that the doctor did not know, but that he did not apply his knowledge fully and assiduously in the interests of the patient. To tell whether the doctor has or has not done so, the patient looks for behavior that, in one combination or another, seems to mean "competence," in the patient's estimate. Some patients rely mainly on indicators that are also evidence of personal interest: respect for the patient's ability to give information, attentiveness, deliberateness, thoroughness, and time taken in obtaining the medical history of the patient and in doing the physical examination. Others with perhaps more experience of illness and medical care look for the presence of specific questions, examinations, or procedures in certain situations: for example, a history of the diet and a patch test when allergy is suspected, or an electrocardiogram when there is chest pain. To some patients, competence, or its use on behalf of the patient, is indicated by a greater quantity of "objective" tests: blood pressure measurements, x-rays, electrocardiograms, laboratory tests. This is especially true when these procedures are covered by a prepayment plan. Within limits, a good doctor will admit uncertainty, but will also take steps to ascertain the true state of affairs by further observation, more tests, and consultation. He will avoid saying, "Do not worry," or "Nothing is wrong," without a sound basis for saying so, as the patient sees it. He will also avoid unpleasant or risky modes of treatment, especially surgery. In general, a good doctor is active; he intervenes if only by naming the illness or prescribing for it. And, finally, the favorable results of his intervention are apparent within some "reasonable" period of time, as perceived by the patient.

In summary, the people studied by Freidson defined quality in terms of certain behaviors on the part of the physician, or attributes of his care, which they felt denoted personal interest or competence. And these two traits were, themselves, interrelated, since they were necessary conditions to a highly individualized application of medical knowledge to each patient's condition, in a manner that took account of the patient's needs, expectations, and preferences. This is, obviously, an "individualized definition" of quality that fits well within the unifying model I described in Chapter One. It does differ, however, in that it does not account for monetary cost, unless by suggesting that when there is prepayment, the use of more tests and procedures is regarded to signify competence. Perhaps more fundamental is the absence of emphasis, in the way clients talk about their doctors, on the relationship between the desirable attributes of the doctor's behavior and its consequences to health and welfare. I believe that this is only an apparent discrepancy, and that from the reported findings one can safely draw the inference that the attributes and behaviors said to be desirable are valued because of their contribution to the patient's welfare.

The attributes of good care identified by Freidson crop up in various combinations in many studies. But his conclusion that personal interest and competence are essentially equal and inseparable categories has not dulled the continuing interest in separating the two, and in finding out which is more important for what kinds of patients. Some information on this subject comes from a study by Cartwright, which has the added interest of telling us about people in another country, under a different system of care (Cartwright 1967, pp.5-9). This is a study of general practice, and the respondents are a probability sample of the inhabitants of England and Wales, who were interviewed in the summer of 1964.

"What are the qualities, the things about your G.P., that you appreciate?" each respondent was asked. The replies, as classified by the investigator, are given in Table 2-1. Of those interviewed, 84 percent mentioned something that they appreciated about the general practitioner's manner or personality, 67 percent something about the way the practitioner looked after the patient; 14 percent mentioned qualities that did not fit exclusively under either of the two previous categories, and 4 percent had only criticisms or could not remember anything particular that they appreciated in their doctors. Respondents were also asked whether there were any other qualities they felt a general practitioner ought to have, but thought theirs did not. Three-quarters of those interviewed could not think of anything, one-fifth had some criticism, and the rest were doubtful or did not know. The respondents who said their doctors were deficient in some way (a fifth of the total) were divided as follows: 6 percent said their doctor was overworked or had too many patients, 5 percent said he did not always listen, 2 percent said he did not go into

Table 2-1

Percent of Respondents Who Mention Specified
Attributes in Answer to the Question "What Are
the Qualities, the Things About Your G.P.,
That You Appreciate?" England and Wales, 1964.

Attributes		*Percent of Respondents*
A. Something about his manner or personality		84
Thoughtful, considerate, sympathetic, or friendly	24	
Approachable or "homely"	18	
More vague characteristics such as pleasant or a very good fellow	15	
Listens, has patience, takes his time	14	
Frank, straightforward, or blunt	12	
Good with children	9	
Gives confidence	6	
Explains things	4	
B. The way he looks after the patient		67
Capable, knows his stuff, good at his job	22	
Visits promptly or without grumbling	19	
Thorough, conscientious	12	
Refers people to the hospital promptly	5	
C. Mixed; related to manner or looking after		14
D. Only criticisms, or could not recall anything particular that was appreciated		4

Source: Cartwright 1967, pp.5-7.

things properly, 5 percent had other criticisms of his manner, and 3 percent gave specific examples of unsatisfactory care.

Perhaps the most striking thing about this study is the finding that such a large proportion of people could think of nothing that was lacking in their doctors. This corresponds to the high levels of satisfaction with medical care found also in the U.S. But these findings, though they give some information about the public's perception of the quality of care, are not germane to the definition of quality itself. With respect to the definition of quality, it is clear that the greater emphasis is on attributes that pertain to the management of the interpersonal relationship, which corresponds to Freidson's category of "personal interest." But I believe that it would be wrong to conclude from the relative frequency of the valued attributes that the quality of technical care is of less importance to people. A more likely explanation is that technical competence is assumed by many to be generally present, so that other characteristics, which obviously vary a great deal from doctor to doctor, become more distinguishing among practitioners.

A U.S. study that is in some respects a counterpart to Cartwright's United Kingdom study is a national survey of an area probability sample of adults that was conducted during the summer of 1955 (Feldman 1966). Among the many questions asked of those interviewed was one that listed nineteen attributes of doctors and invited the respondent to "pick out the four or five which describe the kind of doctor you yourself like best," and then "the four or five that you yourself like least." Unfortunately, besides having a potential confining effect on the range of answers, the list of descriptions Feldman offered included very few items that were directly related to the concept of quality. Moreover, the findings are not fully reported. We are told, however, that 62 percent of the respondents selected the phrase "takes his time" and 56 percent the phrase "very up to date" among the desirable attributes of doctors; and 50 percent selected "old fashioned" among the undesirable attributes. We may infer that the quality of medical care is conceived by many, if not a majority of persons, as technical competence, plus the willingness and the opportunity to use that competence on the patient's behalf.[4]

I cannot refrain from noting, though this is marginal to the definition of quality, that Feldman's survey, as Cartwright's did, recorded a preponderance of satisfaction with the medical care received, even though the interviewers were instructed to give the respondent time to think, and to ask for "even little things" that the respondent was not entirely satisfied with. In spite of such pleading by the interviewers, 89 percent of the respondents said they were "entirely satisfied," and only 11 percent said that they were "not entirely satisfied." Feldman concludes that "the responses can scarcely be interpreted as other than overwhelming satisfaction with the quality of medical care that people have been receiving." (p.85)

The preliminary report of a more recent national survey conducted during the fall of 1975 and the winter of 1976 suggests that things have not changed very much (Robert Wood Johnson Foundation 1978). In this survey, 88 percent reported they were satisfied with their last visit to a doctor and 87 percent were satisfied with the quality of care they had received. Satisfaction was lowest with out-of-pocket cost (60 percent), and next to lowest with time spent waiting to see the doctor (72 percent). But, in spite of these high rates of satisfaction, 61 percent agreed, "There is a crisis in health care today in the United States," 26 percent were uncertain, and only 13 percent disagreed. This remarkable discrepancy remains unexplained. Why, one wonders, is the general view of the medical care world so different from what seems to be warranted by the sum of individual experiences in receiving care?

Turning away from large-scale surveys to more intensive investigations of care received in institutional settings, one finds the remarkable study made by Sussman et al. of the opinions of patients and staff both before and after physical and organizational changes were made in the outpatient clinics of Case Western Reserve University (Sussman et al. 1967). Among other things, patients in the clinics that primarily treat long-term illness were asked early in the study to describe the "good doctor." Attributes of interpersonal and communication skills alone were mentioned by 49.1 percent of patients, whereas 26.6 percent mentioned only technical skills, and 24.3 percent mentioned both (Sussman et al. 1967, Table 3, p.50). These results correspond to the findings of Cartwright in showing an emphasis on the management of the interpersonal process, and to the findings of Coser in revealing two different orientations, even though the findings differ from Coser's in that they imply that there is a much larger "mixed" group. As with Coser's study, the findings of Sussman et al. pertain to a very special institutional setting. The patients of the clinic had long-term illnesses, and were more likely than the general population to be black, female, over 65, unemployed, poor, divorced, widowed, or separated. This means that one must be very cautious in generalizing from these findings. Besides, a somewhat different picture emerged when the patients were asked to assess the clinics and the care they give.

Patients in the clinics that treat mainly patients with long-term illness were shown a checklist of 10 items and asked to name "the three things most important for a good clinic." The results are shown in Table 2-2. They demonstrate the high and equal importance given to a well-trained

The Definition of Quality

doctor and a doctor with whom the patient has a stable relationship. The importance of personal interest and of several of the amenities of care is also noteworthy. Unfortunately, we are not quite certain that what I have called the "quality of technical care" can be equated with the meaning that "well-trained" has for the patient. What is more important, we must wonder why, given three choices, not everyone chose "well-trained doctor" as one of the three.

TABLE 2–2

PERCENT OF PATIENTS IN CLINICS THAT TREAT
MAINLY LONG-TERM PATIENTS WHO SELECTED EACH
OF SPECIFIED FEATURES TO BE INCLUDED AMONG
THE THREE MOST IMPORTANT FOR A GOOD CLINIC.
CASE WESTERN RESERVE UNIVERSITY, CLEVELAND, 1961.

Clinic Features	*Percent of Respondents*
Well-trained doctors	59.2
Seeing the same doctor each visit	59.2
Personal interest of doctor in patient	34.0
Privacy in discussing sickness	32.3
Fair clinic charges	30.1
Short wait for the doctor	27.1
Information from doctors	27.1

Source: Sussman et al. 1967, Table 21, p.92. Reproduced with permission.

Three items on the checklist were chosen by less than 20 percent of patients. These were: good rest rooms, pleasant staff, and comfortable waiting rooms.

Additional information comes from a study of the components and correlates of satisfaction with the clinics and the care they provide.[5] Patients were asked their general opinion of the clinics and, according to their responses, they were classified as follows: 42.8 percent very satisfied, 43.9 percent satisfied, 6.5 percent resigned, 5.5 percent dissatisfied, and 1.3 percent "don't know." They were also asked their opinions of a large number of specific features of the clinic, and the relationship between these opinions and general satisfaction was determined. Multiple regression of 22 variables associated with general satisfaction produced two clusters of factors. The first cluster concerned the "clinic milieu" and comprised the patient's evaluations of the waiting rooms, the waiting room seats, the convenience of the rest rooms, the time spent waiting for the doctor, and total time spent in the clinic on the last visit. The second cluster concerned "treatment aspects of the clinic experience," and comprised the patient's evaluations of the clinic doctor, the physician's personal interest in the patient, the assignment of patients to doctors, and the quality of the clinic's medical care and of the clinic's equipment. It appears that aspects of technical performance and the management of the interpersonal process are gathered into one cluster, as one would have predicted from Freidson's formulation, whereas the amenities of care, as they were called in Chapter One, come together in another cluster. The patients' views of the components of each of the two clusters, when combined into two indexes, are significantly associated with the degree of overall satisfaction, but the treatment cluster has a stronger association with satisfaction. A more detailed view of these associations is obtained by determining the separate effect on overall satisfaction of each of the 22 variables mentioned earlier in this paragraph, using multiple regression analysis. The most important single factor is found to be approval of clinic medical care. The authors conclude that "there is considerable evidence that outpatients place far greater weight on the quality of the medical care than on the surroundings and procedures in arriving at an estimate of the total clinic situation." (Sussman et al. 1967, p.73)

Perhaps one could reasonably say in summary that the clinic population can distinguish the amenities of clinic care from other, more important constituents of its quality; that quality is seen to consist primarily in the use of medical competence in the service of each patient; and that, of the two — competence versus personal commitment — the second is regarded to be the more difficult to come by in the clinic environment.

A similar interpretation may be placed on the findings of another survey of clinic patients, taken at the University of Oklahoma Hospital (Fisher 1971). In this study, patients were given a list of 15 clinic attributes and asked to say whether each was most important, important, or nice for any good clinic. "Good" doctors, well-trained staff, and information from doctors were rated most important.[6] Rated important were personal interest in the patient, pleasant staff, and privacy in discussing illness. Play area for children, convenient food facilities, and a pleasant waiting room were consistently rated low. But, here again, one cannot assume that "good doctor" necessarily means "technical competence," for when patients were asked to describe a "good" doctor, they mentioned "interest in the patient" (personality), "skilled and thorough," and "explains things to you." Moreover, differences in satisfaction with clinic care are correlated with differences in perception of the personal interest shown in the patient, and less so with how much patients feel they have improved or how adequately they feel their condition has been explained to them. Given these ambiguities, it is perhaps best to accept, as Freidson did, that competence and personal interest are equally important and functionally interrelated elements in good care, and to add that the emphasis on one or the other reflects not so much a perception of relative importance as a perception of greater vulnerability in any given situation.

In the studies of clinic populations reviewed above, correlations between satisfaction with specific clinic attributes and overall satisfaction with clinic care were used to indicate the importance accorded to each of a clinic's attributes. An analogous rationale has been used to determine what categories of attributes people use to judge doctors and medical care services, in general (Ware and Snyder 1975). A questionnaire was developed which listed 80 items designed to elicit attitudes about 22 aspects of physician behavior and attributes of the medical care system. The questionnaire was self-administered, at home, by a probability sample of adults who lived in three counties of southern Illinois. This is a population of poor people, older persons, and women. In order to classify the items into more basic categories, the items first were grouped into subsets of items that are highly intercorrelated, though they correlate little across subsets. This reduced the items to 20 "validated dimensions." Next, four factors were identified by factor analysis based on the mean scores of the items in each of the 20 subgroups. These are shown in Table 2-3. Here, not surprisingly, we meet some old friends. Of these, "continuity — convenience," "access," and "availability" would fit under the heading of conditions that are causally related to the quality of care. The items in the remaining factor, "physician conduct," come closer to the core definition of quality that I adopted in Chapter One. They are, in essence, behaviors of the practitioners that are thought to facilitate the attainment of the highest net benefit from care as valued by the fully informed consumer. The authors make much of the fact that the "curing" and "caring" items were not separated by the analysis, but were gathered within one factor. They also note that many of these items also have high loadings on Factors III and IV. This suggests to the authors that "to a certain extent patients generalize their favorable or unfavorable attitudes regarding their physicians and health services characteristics." (p.679)

Somewhat similar findings are reported by Hulka et al., who used a scale that classified its component items into 3 categories: (1) personal qualities of physicians, (2) professional competence, and (3) cost and convenience. In one study, people with generally low income and little

TABLE 2-3

Factors and Their Component Items, Derived
from Analysis of Responses to a Questionnaire
on Attitudes about Doctors and Medical Care
Services. Three Counties in Southern Illinois, 1973.

Factors and Items	*Percent of Common Variance Explained*
I. *Physician Conduct*	30
A. "Curing" function	
Information giving	
Preventive measures	
Thoroughness	
Follow-up care	
Prudence (Discretion)	
B. "Caring" function	
Reassurance	
Consideration of feelings	
Courtesy and respect	
II. *Availability*	21
Having hospitals	
Having specialists	
Having family doctors	
Complete office facilities	
III. *Continuity — Convenience*	24
Continuity of care	
Regular family doctor	
Convenience of services	
IV. *Access*	25
Cost of care	
Emergency care	
Payment mechanisms	
Medical insurance coverage	
Ease of medical check-up	

Source: Ware and Snyder 1975, Table 4, p.677. The "items" in the table are actually clusters of a more detailed listing of 80 questions. I am responsible for assigning each item exclusively to one factor.

education expressed opinions about doctors and the care they had received which showed the three categories of the scale to be significantly correlated with one another, but with apparently greater correlation between opinions about personal qualities and professional competence than between other pairs (Hulka et al. 1971). Subsequent studies of less atypical population groups confirmed the presence of interrelationships among the three categories, but did not show any one pairing to be more closely linked than any other (Zyzanski et al. 1974; Hulka et al. 1975). According to the investigators, "These positive correlations obviously reflect a certain degree of 'halo' effect in that patients with generally favorable attitude toward medical care are likely to generalize these feelings across all components." (Zyzanski et al. 1974, p.619) Nonetheless, it is also likely that some people do actually receive care that is satisfactory across all categories, whereas others receive care that is deficient in most respects.

Much of the work reviewed in this section fits comfortably within the framework I have developed in this book. The "curing" and "caring" functions that are referred to by Ware and Snyder and by Hulka and her coworkers correspond roughly to technical care and the management of the interpersonal process, respectively; and their presence in one factor, though with a kind of halo that spreads out to other factors, fits well with the unifying model for defining quality. It is also in keeping with my interpretation of the literature concerning the relative importance of "competence" and "personal interest," which was summarized earlier in this chapter. The only apparent discrepancy that is important is the discovery of cost in the factor of "access," as demonstrated by Ware and Snyder. But, as the a priori classification of Hulka et al. also shows, this is a legitimate place for cost to be, since cost is an important element in accessibility. It would be unrealistic to expect the method of analysis used by Ware and Snyder to reveal the role that the unifying model assigns to cost in the definition of quality.

The Providers' View of Quality

The providers of care comprise a vast array of policy makers, administrators, supervisors, and practitioners, purveying a great variety of clinical and related services. The literature reviewed in this section deals only with professional practitioners who administer, supervise, or provide direct patient care.

Practitioners tend to define quality not in general terms, but by specifying in detail the clinical activities of patient care, focusing almost exclusively on technical management. A discussion of such specification belongs in a volume on Criteria, which will follow this one. This section will deal with an embarrassingly small number of studies in which the purpose was either to dissect the concept of quality, or to reconstruct the "dimensions" of clinical performance. A little more on the subject will appear in the next section, where I shall compare the opinions of practitioners and clients.

In the preceding section of this chapter we got a view of what patients think makes a good clinic. A corresponding study tells us how health professionals with administrative or supervisory responsibility answer a similar question (Klein et al. 1961). The persons interviewed were 24 "administrative officials in six metropolitan hospitals," among whose number were "out-patient directors of nursing, supervisors, directors of social service, and medical directors." The respondents were asked to think of the best and worst clinics they knew, "in terms of the quality of patient care," and to say what about these clinics made them conclude "this was best" or "this was worst." The result was a list of 80 attributes which the authors classified into 13 categories, as shown in Table 2-4. One can see that administrators and supervisors, perhaps as one might have expected, thought most often of the way the clinic was set up and run. Accordingly, they mentioned features that they believed influence the ability to deliver good care, without, for the most part, identifying the "intrinsic aspects" or "intrinsic ingredients of patient care" that the investigators were looking for, and which we also are trying to find. The omission of the effects of care on "health," as that concept is usually defined, is particularly striking, while patient satisfaction and, to a lesser extent, patient understanding, appear as important characteristics that distinguish the best clinics from the worst. The lesser importance given to "medical skills and facilities" as compared to attributes of personnel and to patient satisfaction is also notable. This is not unlike the relative emphasis placed on the doctor's personal interest by the clients in similar clinics. But, as I pointed out when client opinions were discussed, this inference of relative importance is open to challenge. In this particular study, one could argue that the frequency of mentioning different attributes of the clinics does not represent relative importance as much as it does the discriminating power of each of the attributes. For example, the findings might mean that, in reality, the best and worst clinics differ from each other more often in the degree of concern for patient satisfaction and convenience than in medical skills and facilities. Similarly, it could be that "patient teaching and understanding" is mentioned less frequently than expected either because it is good in all clinics or, more probably, because it is equally bad in all.

TABLE 2-4

THE FREQUENCY WITH WHICH 24 ADMINISTRATORS
AND SUPERVISORS MENTION CLASSES OF ATTRIBUTES
OF OUTPATIENT CLINICS AS DISTINGUISHING
CHARACTERISTICS OF THE "BEST" AND "WORST"
CLINICS THEY HAVE KNOWN. SIX METROPOLITAN
HOSPITALS, BOSTON, CIRCA 1960.

Categories of Attributes	Number of Persons (Total = 24)	Number of Times (Total = 218)
Attitudes of personnel towards patients, doctors, etc.	19	37
Interrole, interdepartmental coordination	17	40
Case loads, amounts of contact with patients	17	38
Patient satisfaction and convenience	15	27
Medical skills and facilities	11	22
Physical facilities	11	11
Continuity of care: same personnel see patient on return visits	9	13
Follow-up: e.g., patients keep return appointments	7	7
Patient teaching and understanding	5	7
Patient–staff relations	4	5
Record system	4	4
Research emphasis	4	4
Staff interpersonal relations	3	3

Source: Klein et al. 1961, Table 1, p.139. Reproduced with permission.

The investigators conclude that there is a large number of attributes of good care, many of which are difficult or impossible to measure; and those that can be measured separately cannot be combined into a "single, comprehensive" measure of patient care. Klein et al. even question whether one can "retain the idea of patient care as a unitary concept," or whether it must remain, similar to the concept of "morale," a bundle of disparate attributes that must be assessed one by one. In Chapter One of this monograph I have argued that a unitary, or unifying, concept of good care can be constructed. I do, however, agree with Klein et al. when they say, "It should be remembered that a concept such as patient care has little 'reality' beyond its usefulness to the scientific or practical ends it is designed to serve. Any definition of the concept is to some extent arbitrary, and in and of itself adds nothing to knowledge unless it serves to further the knowledge-building process." (Klein et al. 1961, p.144)

We may conclude that when one asks a question that is meant to explore the meaning of quality through an indirect route, one gets answers that are in keeping with the professional roles of those questioned, and that are as indirectly related to the concept of quality as was the question. This was true with regard to the answers of administrators and supervisors. A study of the views of physicians shows how those whose primary role is to provide direct patient care respond in an analogous situation (Sanazaro and Williamson 1968a, 1968b, 1970). In this study about 2,500 physicians who were engaged in the full-time private practice of one of several specialties, and who were also faculty members of one of twenty medical schools in 14 states, were asked to describe three episodes of "effective" and three episodes of "ineffective" care that had occurred during the preceding year in the respondent's own practice or had been observed in that of a colleague. The report was to include the specific actions of the physician, the observed or inferred effects on the patient, and an interpretation of what made the performance of the physician "effective" or "ineffective." The method that was used for eliciting information is a "modified version of the critical incident technique,"[7] and the underlying assumption is that practitioners are most likely to view quality in terms of actions that contribute to desired outcomes. It was hoped that the descriptions of "actions" and "effects" in instances of clearly successful care would identify how the physicians themselves defined good or bad performance. This general approach has obvious similarities to the one I used to define quality in Chapter One of this monograph. There, the quality of care was defined in terms of practitioners' decisions and behaviors that were expected to yield the highest net benefit to individuals and to society. It is interesting, therefore, to see how physicians perceive the benefits of care, and what actions they consider to contribute to these benefits.

Of the physicians who were questioned, 94 percent responded, sending in 12,886 descriptions of effective and ineffective care – the former generally episodes in the respondent's own practice, and the latter mainly episodes in the practices of others. One subset of these descriptions was used by the investigators to develop a classification of actions, and another of effects.[8] Table 2-5 shows the major categories of "beneficial" and "detrimental" effects, which the investigators call "end results," that were noted in a subset of incidents reported by internists. Table 2-6 shows the "effective" and "ineffective" actions cited most frequently by internists as causes of "beneficial" and "detrimental" effects, respectively.

TABLE 2-5

FREQUENCY DISTRIBUTION OF INSTANCES OF BENEFICIAL
AND DETRIMENTAL EFFECTS ATTRIBUTED TO PHYSICIAN
ACTIONS, AS REPORTED BY INTERNISTS ENGAGED IN
FULL-TIME PRIVATE PRACTICE WHO WERE ALSO
MEMBERS OF THE FACULTY OF ONE OF TWENTY
MEDICAL SCHOOLS. U.S.A., CIRCA 1965.

Major Categories of Effects	Frequency (Percent)	
	Detailed	Grouped
All Categories	100.0	100.0
Risks	1.8	1.8
Longevity, including mortality	12.3	12.3
Physical abnormalities	20.6 ⎫	
Physical symptoms	15.6 ⎬	40.5
General condition	4.3 ⎭	
Psychological abnormalities	⎫	
Psychological symptoms	⎬	9.3
Function (self-care and social roles)	12.3	12.3
Attitudes toward physician or care	7.8 ⎫	
Attitudes toward condition	5.2 ⎬	18.2
Compliance	5.2 ⎭	
Hospitalization	2.4 ⎫	
Cost	3.2 ⎬	5.6

Source: Sanazaro and Williamson 1968b. The categories have been rearranged to facilitate description in the text.[9] The authors give only the frequency of psychological abnormalities and symptoms combined.

A perusal of Table 2-5 shows that the benefits and harmful effects of care, as seen by internists, can be classified into categories that fit very well with those named in my discussion in Chapter One. These are, roughly speaking, physical function, psychological function, social function, client attitudes and behavior relevant to care, and monetary cost. Of course, it is difficult to say to what extent this happy coincidence is the result of the investigators' imposition of a preconceived order on the detailed accounts of the respondents. It is also unclear what inferences can be drawn from the relative frequencies with which the several categories are cited. One possible interpretation is that even well-informed internists tend to place preponderant emphasis on physical health, and are much less mindful of psychological and social functions as critical indicators of success or failure in performance. If longevity is added to physical abnormalities and symptoms, these categories account for almost 53 percent of all the beneficial and detrimental effects cited. Client attitudes and behaviors are the next largest cluster of categories, accounting for 18.2 percent of effects. Monetary cost, which includes the avoidance of hospitalization or its unnecessary use, occupies a very low position, contrary to the attention it enjoys in the definition of quality that is presented in Chapter One of this monograph. This could mean that monetary cost is usually ignored despite its importance to the client, or that, most of the time, cost is not a very important consideration, especially when a great deal of it is covered by health insurance. But the greatest discrepancy between this picture and our model is the infrequency with which "risk" appears in the reports of the effects of care. This could mean that physicians are unable to estimate risk, or that they pay more attention to immediate outcomes than to future prospects. Most probably it means that physicians did not consider an increase or diminution in risk as "hard" enough evidence to cite in their accounts of effective and ineffective performance. Thus, we get reports of the actual consequences of care rather than of the expectations of these consequences.

As to the actions that led to these consequences, physicians report the traditional activities that make up the process of care. As shown in Table 2-6, the great majority of these pertain to the technical procedures involved in taking a history, doing a physical examination, ordering or performing laboratory tests and other examinations, and prescribing or carrying out a variety of treatments. Using a rather generous interpretation, I estimate that about 20 percent of the activities described in a subset of internists' reports pertain to the management of the interpersonal process, and another 10 percent to access, coordination, and the continuity of care. As was true of the distribution of effects, we cannot assert that the relative frequencies of reporting the different types of actions reflect accurately their relative importance in care as perceived by internists. Perhaps the need to report instances of specific actions that were clearly related to concrete outcomes has influenced the picture. But I believe that this picture is not too unlike medical practice in reality. We have also seen that it accommodates rather comfortably, though not precisely, the model of quality that I presented in Chapter One.

TABLE 2-6

FREQUENCY DISTRIBUTION OF ACTIONS THAT ARE
RESPONSIBLE FOR BENEFICIAL AND DETRIMENTAL
EFFECTS OF CARE, AS REPORTED BY INTERNISTS
ENGAGED IN FULL-TIME PRIVATE PRACTICE WHO
WERE ALSO MEMBERS OF THE FACULTY OF ONE OF
TWENTY MEDICAL SCHOOLS. U.S.A., CIRCA 1965.

Categories of Action	Percent of Actions	
	Detailed	Grouped
All Categories	100.1	100.1
Management of the Interpersonal Relationship		20.5
Professional responsibility	4.5	
Professional manner	3.9	
Psychological perception	2.6	
Psychological support	2.9	
Patient education	6.6	
Access, Continuity, Coordination		9.7
Availability of physician	3.3	
Use of health team	0.9	
Use of community resources	0.3	
Review of problem	2.5	
Review of treatment	0.6	
Follow-up	2.1	
Regulation of Diet and Activity	1.7	1.7
Other: Almost Entirely Technical	68.2	68.2

Source: Sanazaro and Williamson 1968a, Table 2, p.394. I am responsible for grouping the categories as they appear in this Table.

In the two studies reviewed so far in this section (Klein et al. and Sanazaro and Williamson) the investigators used a conceptual framework that they themselves provided to classify the opinions and reports of their respondents. We now turn to two studies that used statistical methods to search for affinities among components of care as a basis for grouping them into categories. The first of these, by Hopkins and his associates (1975), offers, in addition, a comparison between two classifications, one constructed without benefit of immediate empirical information, and the other based on the analysis of empirical data.

The impetus for this study was the need to compare the content of care and, if possible, its quality when care was received by subscribers of different types of health insurance plans, including prepaid group practice. As a first step, the quality of care was postulated to have five components, which the authors called "dimensions." Under each of these headings the authors listed specified attributes and elements of care, 36 in all, about which information was likely to be present in the patient's medical record. The "dimensions" and their constituents are listed in Table 2-7. One notes immediately the heavy emphasis on technical care (under the headings of "prevention" and "rationality") and the absence of corresponding attention to the management of the interpersonal relationship. No doubt this reflects the known limitation of the range of information in the medical record.

The next step in this study was to compile for each person in a sample of 805 families a record of ambulatory and inpatient care received during a twelve-month period. The 1,215 records assembled in this way were then physically cut up into segments (called "bits"), each of which contained information about "a single patient-physician encounter and its associated laboratory, radiology, and other ancillary services." The recorded content of the resulting 11,379 bits was then coded to show which of 32 elements of care (of the original 36) were included. Some items were simply coded as present or absent. Others were scored with the use of a Lickert-type scale. For example, the physical examination was scaled as scanty, full, or detailed. The replicability of scoring received careful attention, and while there may have been many imperfections in the method, the authors believe that, in the end, "a significant step had been achieved in making possible objective statistical analysis of data obtainable from medical records."

The third step in the procedure was to reduce the thirty-odd items that described the attributes and elements of care into a smaller set by the use of factor analysis with varimax rotation. After two reiterations, 20 items were kept: 15 because of highly significant loadings on one of the first four factors, and another 5 because they seemed to have conceptual sig-

TABLE 2-7

AN INITIAL CLASSIFICATION OF THE CONTENT OF
MEDICAL CARE COMPARED TO A CLASSIFICATION
THAT EMERGED FROM FACTOR ANALYSIS OF THE
CONTENT OF CARE RECEIVED BY A SAMPLE OF
FAMILIES ENROLLED IN SELECTED HEALTH
INSURANCE PLANS. LOS ANGELES, CIRCA 1970.

"Dimensions" *Postulated* *Initially*	*Attributes or Elements of* *Care Postulated Initially* *To Belong in Each* *"Dimension"*	*Items Retained* *by Preliminary* *Factor Analysis*	*Prevention*	*Continuity*	*Rationality*	*Verification*
			Factors Finally Identified			
Prevention	Check-up examination	X	X			
	Rectal examination	X	X			
	Pelvic examination	X	X			
	Papanicolaou smear	X	X			
	Chest x-ray	X				X
	Prenatal check-up	–				
	Immunization	X				
	Well-baby examination	–				
	Serology	X				X
	Advice on avoidance of future problems	–				
Comprehensiveness	Secondary conditions found, etc.	–				
	Social factors	X				
Coordination	Referral: specialist	X				
	Referral: paramedic	–				
	Consultation services	–				
Continuity	Follow-up visit	X		X		
	Follow-up visit requested	X		X		
	Continuity of medical personnel	X				
	Continuity of medical record	–				
	Progress notes	X			X	
	Rehabilitation Services	–				

TABLE 2-7 — *Continued*

"Dimensions" Postulated Initially	*Attributes or Elements of Care Postulated Initially To Belong in Each "Dimension"*	*Items Retained by Preliminary Factor Analysis*	Factors Finally Identified			
			Prevention	*Continuity*	*Rationality*	*Verification*
Rationality	Chief complaint	X			X	
	History	X			X	
	Physical examination	X	X		X	
	Diagnosis	X			X	
	Laboratory work ordered	—				
	Laboratory results recorded	X				
	Physician seen	—				
	Surgery (amount)	—				
	Treatment: injection	—				
	Treatment: prescription	—				
	Treatment: other	—				
	Complete blood count	X				X
	Urinalysis	X				X
	Other laboratory work (amount)	—				
	Other radiology (amount)	—				

Source: Hopkins et al. 1975, Tables 1 and 2, pp.200, 203.

nificance. The third column of Table 2-7 shows which items were dropped and which remained.

As a fourth step, factor analysis was repeated with the smaller set of 20 items. The result was the identification of four factors, which are also shown in the Table. Of the original five dimensions, two, "comprehensiveness" and "coordination," were lost. Of the remaining three dimensions, "prevention" and "continuity" remained as important factors, while "rationality" was split into two factors that were named "rationality" and "verification." The resulting four factors explain 42 percent of the variance among cases; "prevention" accounts for 17.5 percent of the variance, "continuity" for 7.5 percent, "rationality" for 9.5 percent, and "verification" for 7.9 percent. The most important attributes and elements of care that constitute each factor are shown in Table 2-7.

The investigators go on to show that it is possible (by using as weights the loadings of each item on each factor, and the percentage of variance explained by each factor) to construct scores that permit comparisons among plans by each factor separately, and by all factors combined. This appears to be a reasonable method for eliciting differences in the actual content of care. But it is not clear to what extent these are also differences in quality. The question is raised because the content of care depends heavily on case mix; the weighting of the components of care does not necessarily correspond to the benefits they are expected to yield; and the appropriateness of care has not been determined, unless the assumption has been made that all the procedures are appropriate in all cases. I agree, however, with the investigators in their concluding that the method deserves further study as a means for assessing the quality of care.

An assessment of whether the method is also a superior means for specifying the meaning of "the quality of care" as a concept is closer to our interests in this chapter. I have already referred to an important weakness in the data: the medical record does not show all that has been done for the patient, and it certainly does not show all that should have been done. As to the interpretation of the factors themselves, this depends on the nature of the items that are subjected to factoring, and of the basis for the patterns of association among these items. In this particular case, these items are mainly components of care rather than components of "goodness." It is not clear what accounts for the associations among items, but these are likely to be determined partly by the types of cases that are presented for care, and partly by the methods of management selected by the physician. Consequently, the factors identified by analysis can be nothing more than distinguishable categories of care that are set apart because they serve separable functions in particular types of cases. For example, yearly check-ups call for a particular set of "case-finding" examinations which are not, in practice, often done in other cases, even though they probably should be done more frequently. Similarly, the management of illness seems to involve two clusters or "packages" of care. One of these includes the history, the physical examination, and the recording of progress notes and diagnosis, and the other is made up of a bundle of diagnostic tests. In this instance, the factor analysis has been useful in separating these two clusterings, even though their components were originally combined under the misleading rubric of "rationality." I would guess that the first of these factors denotes not "rationality," but a tendency to keep more complete records, whereas the second factor shows reliance on diagnostic testing in the management of illness.

The factor analysis has also revealed that chest x-rays and "serology" are generally part of the battery of diagnostic tests (the factor of "verification") rather than part of the preventive set, as it was originally proposed. I do not believe this means that chest x-rays and serology are not used preventively. It is more likely that the original classification, and the coding based on it, did not provide for a distinction between preventive and diagnostic use of these items, as it should have done. The loss of the two categories of "comprehensiveness" and "coordination" as a result of factor analysis may mean that these attributes are lacking in medicine as it is actually practiced. I prefer to believe that these attributes were not identified because they were not appropriately conceptualized and measured. If this is the case, the factor analysis has served to point out these deficiencies. It is more difficult to justify the early elimination of prenatal check-ups and well-baby examinations, among the items that were "redundant or meaningless," and the nonappearance of "immunizations" in the factor of prevention, even though immunizations made the final list of the elements of care. On the basis of these observations I am inclined to see factor analysis as a method for checking on, and refining, the original classification, rather than as a substitute.

In discussing the preceding study I emphasized that case mix and the appropriateness of care were ignored. Both of these factors were addressed in another study, where factor analysis was also used to identify the dimensions of care. This is a study of the quality of ambulatory care by Riedel and Riedel (1979). In order to assess quality, panels of physicians specified the elements of care, called "criteria," that should be present in the management of each of nine conditions identified either by diagnosis or by major presenting symptom. The criteria pertain almost exclusively to technical care, excluding the management of the interpersonal process. Adherence to these criteria was determined primarily by review of the records of ambulatory care, which means that the findings reflect patterns of performance and of recording combined.

The quality of performance is defined as the degree of adherence to the "criteria" of care. Since adherence varied widely from criterion to criterion, and the number of criteria was very large, factor analysis is used to reveal underlying patterns in physician performance. The object is to identify categories of criteria (signifying areas of care) that are similar to one another with respect to adherence, but unrelated to other categories in this respect. What emerges, as shown in Table 2-8, is a bewildering variety of groupings that differ considerably from condition to condition. Although certain factors such as "history," "physical examination," and "laboratory" appear repeatedly, there are many factors that are highly specific to each condition. Thus, it was not possible, with this method, to develop a classification that organizes performance in a general sense. Moreover, it is often difficult even to guess what processes account for the association of several items of performance in any given factor. For example, it is rather easy to understand why, in the management of adult abdominal pain, elements such as "abdominal rebound," "abdominal guarding," "abdominal tenderness," and "abdominal masses" should cohere into one factor. These are, after all, functionally related elements of a reasonably thorough examination of the abdomen, so that if one element is performed the others are also likely to be performed, and if the findings of one are recorded many of the others are also likely to be recorded in what is almost a litany, learned by repeated practice. But what, one wonders, can account for the grouping into one factor, in the same condition, of the following elements: "constant pain, persistent pain, onset of pain, affecting factors, food and drugs, working diagnosis, pulse, blood pressure, pelvic exam, relationship of mensis to pain, temperature, and chest exam"? Of course, one could speculate. For example, awareness of the importance of the attributes of pain should lead to a cluster of related questions concerning pain, but one finds that not all the attributes of the pain are included in this factor. Several remain in a "residual" category. Pelvic examination and the question about menstrual pain are a reasonably linked pair. Similarly, pulse, blood pressure, and temperature could denote attention to recording the vital signs. But what does this have to do with the gynecological dyad, with emphasis on the attributes of pain, with doing a chest examination, or with recording a working diagnosis? Many of the factors appear to have a similar structure, lending themselves to subdivision into smaller functionally related clusters. I am not sure what this means, but it does suggest that a more careful, more clinically informed reassessment of the data might result in a more satisfactory mapping of the structure of clinical performance than is provided by the factors as they now stand. Even if a more meaningful classification were to emerge, it would identify elements of technical performance concerning which judgments of quality have to be made; it would not improve our understanding of the concept of quality. This is

TABLE 2-8

FACTORS IDENTIFIED BY FACTOR ANALYSIS OF
FINDINGS ON COMPLIANCE WITH EXPLICIT CRITERIA
IN A STUDY OF RECORDED AMBULATORY CARE OF
SPECIFIED CONDITIONS. HARTFORD AND NEW HAVEN,
CONNECTICUT, 1974–1975.

Abdominal Pain, Adult
Abdomen
Bowel movement
Nausea
Diagnosis
History
Lab

Pediatric Abdominal Pain
Physical exam
Vomiting
Ingestion
Lab

Chest Pain
Physical exam
History
Symptom 1
Symptom 2
Follow–up

Hypertension
General follow–up
First visit
Follow–up eye exam
First lab
Initial eye exam
Family history
Blood pressure check
Basics

Urinary Infection
Pain
Previous treatment
Lab
Diagnosis
Severe

Pharyngitis
Instructions
Diagnosis
Throat exam
Ear exam

Otitis media
Treatment
Follow–up 1
Follow–up 2
Disease
History

Well Child (Infant)
Physical exam
Development
Birth
Follow–up
Family
Size

Well Child (Preschool)
Physical exam
History
Follow–up
Size

Source: Riedel and Riedel 1979. In each of the conditions there is a "residual category" which is not included in the Table. See Tables 7.2a–7.10a, pages 130–39 of the source.

because the analysis as a whole begins with a fundamental assumption that is not subject to testing: that the quality of care is a form of normative behavior which is manifested through adherence to professional dicta.

Comparisons of the Views of Clients and Providers

Something more about how clients and providers perceive the quality of care can be learned from studies that have expressly compared the two viewpoints. One of these is a part of a long series devoted to the measurement and prediction of physician performance (Price et al. 1964, 1971). The basic concern that led to this long-lasting effort was the proper selection of medical students. Earlier studies had shown that the grades of undergraduates do predict grades in medical school, but that neither undergraduate grades nor grades in medical school predict performance in practice. But this conclusion was open to challenge because the dependent variable, "performance in practice," had not been measured well. Recognizing the critical nature of this defect, a group of investigators at the University of Utah set out to develop better measures of physician performance, and to test the ability of grades and other variables to predict performance. In their earlier studies the investigators say that they "purposely avoided direct work on the highly sensitive area of patient care." Accordingly, I shall not describe the earlier measures of success in a medical career that they developed. More relevant are the findings of a later study in which the investigators believed that they were dealing with "the very heart of physician performance – the quality of service given to patients." (Price et al. 1971, pp.48ff.)

To help them find their way to this innermost shrine the investigators asked a large number of physicians the following question: "With regard to your field of specialty, what do you consider to be the basic factors of success?" Answers from 372 physicians were compiled in a list which was then submitted to "over 100 selected, thoughtful individuals – medical educators, college and medical students, and patients recuperating in, or recently discharged from hospitals." Guided by the comments of this second group, the investigators developed a final list of 87 "desirable" and 29 "undesirable" attributes. The next step was to submit the two revised lists to a variety of people who were asked to rate each attribute on a five-point scale as to "importance to superior physician performance" or "detrimentality to superior physician performance," depending on whether the attribute was a desirable or an undesirable one. The average scores were then used to rank the attributes.

In all, ten groups of people rated the attributes. These groups are described as (1) general public, up to age 65, (2) general public, age 65 and over, (3) practicing physicians, (4) medical students, interns, and residents, (5) nurses, (6) medical technicians, (7) college students, (8) "lower socioeconomic group," (9) "hippies," and (10) "blacks." It is not clear how these respondents were selected, but we are told that "a portion of the data for this group was gathered in the redemption centers of a large trading company. . . . Other data were obtained by personal contact or by mail." This procedure raises some doubts about the degree to which one may safely generalize from this sample. But an even more important defect is that the questions asked do not seem to specify "patient care" or "quality." Instead, the authors of the report use expressions like "success" or "superior performance."

In spite of these limitations, it seemed to me that one could learn something by comparing the rankings of the different physician attributes by different groups of respondents. Figure 2-1 is a scatter diagram of the rankings by two groups: the general public and physicians. The Spearman rank correlation coefficient is 0.83 for the desirable attributes and 0.88 for the undesirable ones. The ratings of nurses agree at least as well with those of the general public, the corresponding coefficients being 0.91 and 0.93 respectively.[10]

Table 2-9 gives a more detailed look at the top ten attributes as ranked by physicians and the general public, respectively. Of these, seven attributes are shared, and the discrepancy is small in an additional two. Both parties agree on the preeminent importance of knowledge, judgment, thorough examination, and an appropriate recognition by the physician of his own limitations, as shown by a readiness to refer patients when this is needed. I consider all these to be aspects of the responsible exercise of a high level of clinical competence. Beyond this area of virtual agreement, physicians, apparently more aware of their own limitations, put greater emphasis on intellectual honesty and on the ability to continue to learn. Members of the general public place the greatest weight on knowledge already acquired, on the maintenance of clinical records, and on the ability to inspire confidence in patients. A perusal of the remaining items, beyond the top ten in each ranking, suggests that the public places greater relative importance on attributes that connote competence and the ability to work with patients, while physicians emphasize the capacity to work hard and to get along with colleagues.

The degree of agreement on undesirable attributes is even greater than that on the desirable ones. Of the five attributes ranked most undesirable by physicians, all are among the worst five as ranked by the general public; but this degree of agreement is partly the result of the listing of very serious defects such as alcoholism and drug addiction among the undesirable attributes that were rated.

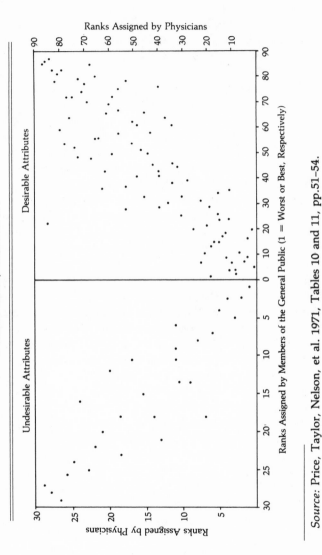

FIGURE 2-1

DESIRABLE AND UNDESIRABLE ATTRIBUTES OF PHYSICIANS RELATED TO THEIR
PROFESSIONAL PERFORMANCE, RANKED ACCORDING TO RATINGS OF EACH ATTRIBUTE
BY SELECTED GROUPS OF PRACTICING PHYSICIANS AND BY MEMBERS OF THE GENERAL
PUBLIC. UTAH, CIRCA 1969.

Source: Price, Taylor, Nelson, et al. 1971, Tables 10 and 11, pp.51-54.

A summary, by its very nature, must ignore a great deal of detailed information that may be important; but in this instance it seems safe to conclude that there is broad agreement among clients and practitioners about the meaning of good physician performance. Although clients place somewhat greater importance on the physician's ability to relate to patients, and physicians on their ability to work smoothly with colleagues, both agree that the most important thing is a high level of clinical competence exercised in a responsible manner. But more evidence should be examined before this conclusion is accepted as generally applicable.

Some additional information on the similarity of the views of providers and of clients comes from a study of outpatient care which I mentioned earlier in this chapter (Sussman et al. 1967). In this instance, a list of clinic features was submitted to the physicians, nurses, social workers, and secretaries who worked in a clinic, with the request that they rate the importance of each feature to patient care as they themselves saw it, and also its importance to the patient as they perceived the patient's opinions to be. At the same time, patients were asked to say which of the same features they considered to be important to patient care.

The data provided by the investigators allow for a large number of interesting comparisons which are, however, extremely difficult to grasp and describe. To simplify matters a little, I have constructed Figure 2-2, taking the liberty of presenting as a continuous variable something that, obviously, is not. I refer to the several clinic features which are placed on the abscissa in order of diminishing importance in the opinion of physicians. The left-hand panel of Figure 2-2 shows that physicians have a very highly differentiated view of the importance of clinic features, rating some features very high and others very low. By contrast, patients are less discriminating, in that they regard all the features as rather important. Nonphysician clinic staff are in between, but closer to the physicians in this regard. A second finding is that there is considerable agreement about the importance of some features, notably "pleasant staff," "privacy in discussing illness," and "same physician in each illness." Physicians and patients disagree rather widely on all the remaining features, whereas valuations of the nonphysician clinic staff are in some respects closer to those of the patients, and in others closer to those of the physicians, and in still others somewhere in between.

The right-hand panel of Figure 2-2 is of particular interest because it shows a comparison of the patients' actual opinions with the perceptions that others have of those opinions. It appears that, in a very rough way, those who provide care understand what their patients want. But when these results are viewed in detail, there are some interesting discrepan-

TABLE 2–9

DESIRABLE ATTRIBUTES OF PHYSICIANS RANKED
AMONG THE TOP TEN ACCORDING TO THEIR
IMPORTANCE TO SUPERIOR PERFORMANCE, AS
PERCEIVED BY PHYSICIANS AND MEMBERS OF THE
GENERAL PUBLIC. UTAH, CIRCA 1969.

A. Attributes among the Top Ten as Ranked by Both Physicians and the General Public*	Rank by Physicians	Rank by Public
Good clinical judgment (the ability to reach appropriate decisions regarding the care of patients)	1	5
Wise, thoughtful, able to get to the heart of a problem; able to separate important points from details	6	3.5
Knowledge and ability to study patients thoroughly, and to reach sound conclusions regarding diagnosis, treatment, and related problems	8.5	2
Readily refers patients when it is to their advantage to do so	3.5	8.5
Keeps completely honest records	8.5	3.5
Habitually makes as thorough an examination of each patient as may be required for accurate diagnosis and proper treatment	10	6.5
Provides treatment appropriate to condition of each of his patients with (in general) satisfactory results	7	10.5
B. Attributes among the Top Ten as Ranked by Physicians*		
Able to be his own teacher: to learn from books and journals, from meetings and informal discussions, from experience and his own mistakes, etc., thus adding continually to his own education	2.0	19.5

TABLE 2-9 — *Continued*

	Rank by Physicians	Rank by Public
Intellectual honesty (incompatible with bluffing, cheating, assuming poses for ulterior purposes, trickery, claiming undue credit, assuming knowledge not really possessed, transferring blame unfairly, etc.), forthrightness	3.5	16
Able to convert acquired information into working knowledge	5	12

C. Attributes among the Top Ten as Ranked by Members of the General Public*

	Rank by Physicians	Rank by Public
Thorough up-to-date knowledge of his own field of medicine	18.5	1
Keeps full and accurate clinical records	22.5	6.5
Strict about honoring confidences; avoids and discourages gossip	12.5	8.5
Inspires confidence in his patients	21	10.5

Source: Price et al. 1971, Table 10, pp.51–53.

*The attributes among the top ten as ranked by both parties are listed in ascending order of the sum of both ranks. The other attributes are listed in descending order of importance to physicians and to the general public, respectively.

cies. For example, the clinic staff overestimate the importance that the patients place on "seeing the same physician on each visit" and on a "short wait for the physician." On the other hand, they underestimate the importance of "patient knowledge of his condition," "convenient location of clinic services," and "food facilities" at the clinic.

FIGURE 2-2

PERCENT OF SPECIFIED RESPONDENTS WHO EXPRESS SPECIFIED OPINIONS
ABOUT THE IMPORTANCE OF SPECIFIED FEATURES OF THE OUTPATIENT
CLINIC. CASE WESTERN RESERVE UNIVERSITY, CLEVELAND, 1960.

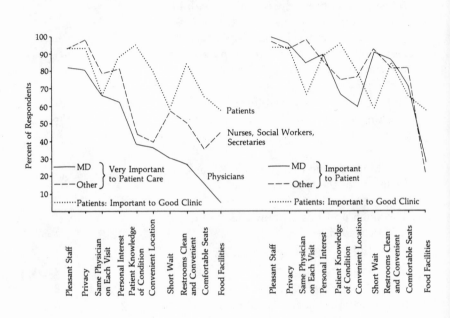

Source: Sussman et al. 1967, Table 40, p.129.

In addition to these comparisons, it would be interesting to know who
is "closer" to the patients: physicians or nonphysician clinic staff. In this
case, nonphysicians are more often more similar to the patients in their
ratings of clinic features, but more often less knowledgeable about the
patients' opinions. Stated another way, the physicians are more different
from patients, but they know the patients better. But these differences are
very small, and could have occurred by chance. Moreover, the inclusion
of secretaries with nurses and social workers virtually invalidates the
comparison of this group with physicians. Finally, it should be noted
that the attributes selected for rating do not include aspects of technical

management, so that nothing can be said about the relative importance of the two larger domains: competence and personal interest. In my opinion, the most noteworthy findings of this study are that the patients' views of what is important in clinic care are more inclusive and less sharply focused than those of the professionals; and that professionals may underestimate the needs of the patients to know about their conditions, while they may overestimate the importance of seeing the same physician, when the institutional setting itself provides reasonable continuity in care. Of course, the generality of these inferences is further limited by the nature of both this particular setting and the population it serves.

Additional information about different views of quality, including the importance of the technical aspects of care compared to other aspects, comes from a study by Smith and Metzner (1970). The locale is a hospital-based prepaid group practice in Detroit. A questionnaire was administered to physicians, nurses, and two samples of male patients who were between 21 and 65 in age; one group consisted of nonemergency, walk-in patients, and the other of patients who had been in the hospital for more than five days. The questionnaire contained two sets of items, as follows: Set One, (a) scientific knowledge: the specific scientific knowledge needed; (b) personal interest: explaining things and showing a personal concern for the patient; (c) cooperation: close teamwork and lack of personal conflicts between those providing care; Set Two, (a) technical skill: the particular technical skills needed; (b) patient comfort: having pleasant surroundings and services that add to the patient's comfort; (c) efficiency: efficiently organized services so that there is little delay in providing what is needed. Respondents were asked to rank the three items in each set separately. Walk-in patients and hospital patients answered for themselves. Physicians and nurses answered having in mind, first, persons similar to the sample of walk-in patients and, then, persons similar to the sample of hospital patients. A portion of the findings is shown in Figure 2-3.

The investigators had intended pairs of attributes in the two triads to be similar in representing three aspects of quality: "a. the technical process, b. the therapeutic relationship existing between the patient and the hospital, and c. the organizational effectiveness of the hospital as a whole." (p.265) The configuration of responses, depicted in Figure 2-3, and a more rigorous analysis by the investigators show that this is not the case. It follows that the findings respecting the two sets of attributes must be interpreted separately. Another finding is that the kind of patient makes a difference in the relative rankings of attributes, especially when

The Definition of Quality

FIGURE 2-3

PERCENT OF RESPONDENTS WHO ASSIGN FIRST RANK
TO SPECIFIED ATTRIBUTES OF GOOD CARE IN EACH OF
TWO TRIADS OF SUCH ATTRIBUTES, BY SITE OF CARE.
A PREPAID GROUP PRACTICE PLAN, DETROIT,
MICHIGAN, CIRCA 1968.

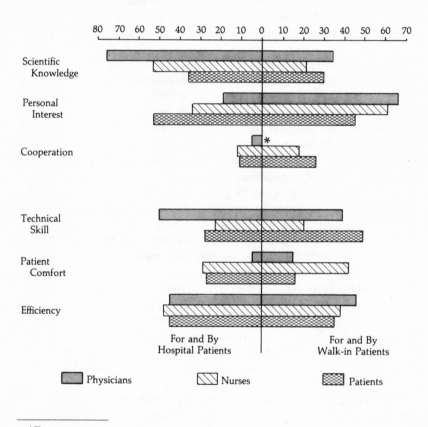

*Zero percent.
Source: Smith and Metzner 1970, Tables 8–11, pp. 271–74.

physicians and nurses are the judges. And finally, the three groups of
respondents differ from one another in their views, the larger difference
being that between the patients and the two groups of professionals combined. In greater detail, the findings for the first triad of attributes rated

by and for walk-in patients show that "explaining things and personal concern for the patient" is most often regarded to be the most important attribute, with scientific knowledge clearly in second place; and, contrary to expectation, physicians and nurses place even more emphasis on personal interest than do the patients, and patients place no less emphasis on scientific knowledge than do the professionals. For hospital patients the picture is different. Patients continue to place the greatest emphasis on personal interest, which stands for explaining and concern, whereas the professionals, and in particular physicians, tilt heavily in favor of scientific knowledge, presumably because the condition of the patient demands it.

An examination of the rankings of the second triad of attributes by and for walk-in patients shows that patients and physicians are in agreement on the primary importance of technical skill and the subsidiary standing of patient comfort, whereas nurses reverse this order, placing the greatest importance on patient comfort and emphasizing this aspect of care much more than the patients do themselves. The rankings by and for hospital patients show that physicians are even more concerned with technical skill and less concerned about patient comfort for this category of patients than for walk-in patients, while nurses and patients divide their attention about equally between technical skill and patient comfort. Of the two attributes of organizational effectiveness, "cooperation" appears to have little importance to physicians in either setting, and it has some importance to nurses and physicians in both settings. By contrast, efficiency, which in this case means expeditious care, is of considerable importance in both settings, often taking precedence over patient comfort.

I wish a clearer summary of this study were possible; but the account I have given already involves greater simplification than is perhaps warranted by the original data and their analysis. In any event, the study shows how difficult it is to specify the ingredients of quality in unequivocal terms. It also demonstrates that the relative importance given to the several ingredients varies not only according to the respondent's role, but also according to the gravity and technical demands of the patient's condition.

Summary and Conclusions

It is very risky to pull together very different studies of rather distinctive populations into one unifying construct; but the mind rebels at so much unorganized variety and demands some synthesis, no matter how crude or fragile that may be. I will, therefore, attempt a summary, not in order to provide definitive conclusions, but as a way of sharing with the reader my own interpretations and impressions.

From the very start we need to realize that investigators who have designed empirical studies of the meaning of quality have generally approached the subject through indirection, by asking about the desirable properties of doctors or clinics, or by identifying the attributes of doctors and clinics that correlate with expressed satisfaction or dissatisfaction with these providers. By these indirect means we seem to get correspondingly indirect answers, which vary according to the role of the respondent. Administrators tend to speak of the way in which a clinic is set up and run. Physicians describe the elements of care, generally placing emphasis on its technical components. Patients describe the amenities of a clinic, and how physicians behave as they interact with them. The mass of resulting details has been reduced and organized in some cases with the use of factor analysis, but more often by a process of sorting out according to conceptual categories that are already present in the investigator's mind. My impression is that factor analysis, where it has been used, has not proved very revealing. It seems to be most useful as an adjunct to conceptual exploration, rather than as a replacement or a primary tool.

In almost all the studies that I have reviewed, quality is defined not in terms of the consequences of care but in terms of attributes of the providers and of their behavior. It seems that consideration of outcomes must be intentionally made part of the study design, if the outcomes are to emerge explicitly as a factor of importance. Nevertheless, we must assume that the expectation of desirable outcomes is the most powerful force that shapes the choice of the desirable attributes of the providers of care, though it is often submerged.

In studies of what clients think makes a good doctor or a good clinic, it is possible to discern three large categories of attributes pertaining, respectively, to the amenities of the settings of care, to aspects of the personal interaction with practitioners, and to technical competence. The first of these, though important to clients, tends to be subsidiary to the other two in relative importance; but the importance of the remaining two categories relative to each other remains undecided. There is some evidence that some people place primary emphasis on the affectual elements of the interpersonal process, whereas others place primary emphasis on the technical elements of care. But I believe that it is closer to reality to say, as Freidson says, that most people want both "personal interest" and "competence." In fact, there is reason to believe that personal interest and competence are an inseparable pair of functionally related clusters of attributes, in that personal interest provides assurance that the competence a physician can command will be used on the patient's behalf.

In spite of the functional linkage between personal interest and competence, people do vary in the relative importance they place on one of the two attributes relative to the other. Perhaps the most plausible explanation is that the relative emphasis depends on which of the two attributes is more likely to be deficient, and on which deficiency is more likely to be damaging to the patient, taking into account the nature of the medical problem. In this light, the greater emphasis placed on aspects of interpersonal management in several of the studies reviewed suggests that many people assume a lesser variation in the technical quality of care, and a greater variability in attributes denoting personal interest. Nevertheless, we must also be ready to find that there are some people who derive more than the usual gratification from personal interest itself.

Analysis of the practice of physicians, as reported in the medical records of care, cannot be expected to give a full picture of the considerations that enter the physician's definition of quality. Many of the things the physician does are not in the record; in particular, information about the management of the interpersonal process is likely to be missing. But when physicians are asked to describe what they consider to be effective or ineffective care, we can infer from their answers a broad definition of health that includes physical function, psychological function, and social function, and a correspondingly broad range of activities that improve or damage these aspects of function. Within this extensive domain, however, there is a clear tendency to emphasize technical management and its impact on physiological health and function.

Comparisons of the viewpoints of clients and practitioners suggest that there is a great deal of similarity between the two. The responsible exercise of technical competence occupies a core position in both. Clients do seem to place somewhat greater relative emphasis on aspects of the interpersonal relationship, and distinctly greater emphasis on the amenities of care than do the practitioners. One suspects that clients have a less clearly differentiated view of the relative importance of the different attributes of care, considering many to be of roughly similar importance. By contrast, physicians appear to have in mind a more sharply ordered hierarchy, and one that is more finely adjusted to suit the nature of the patient's medical problem. This means that, paradoxically, in certain situations physicians would place less emphasis on technical care and more emphasis on personal interest than the patient would. There is also reason to believe that physicians are aware of the patients' preferences, at least in a rough way. At the same time we can find important discrepancies between what patients want and what physicians think the patients want. This means that problems might arise partly because physicians misperceive what patients want, and partly because they cannot, or do not wish to, respond to what they correctly perceive patients to prefer. But, whatever these tensions may be, it is clear that they are contained and counterbalanced by broad agreement on the fundamentals. It must be this that provides stability to the system, and accounts for the high levels of satisfaction with care that are so often reported by clients.

Finally, we must confront the assertion that the attributes of good care, or of a good doctor or a good clinic, are so many and so varied that it is impossible to derive from them either a unifying concept or a single empirical measure of quality. As a corollary, it would be unrealistic to expect that the performance of any one practitioner, or of an institution as a whole, would be so uniform across these many ingredients of quality that the goodness of one aspect would signal the presence of goodness in many of the others also. This is an issue that will concern us deeply as we go on. But, in the meantime, it seems to me that the conceptual model of quality that I presented in Chapter One can rather easily accommodate the empirical findings in all their variety. I hope this does not mean that the model is presented in such general terms that it has no analytic usefulness. I wish that the capacity of the model to accommodate the empirical findings also meant independent confirmation of its validity. Clearly, this is not the case, because I developed the model after the event, when I had the empirical findings already in mind.

Notes to Chapter Two

[1] I have surmised that the question asked by Freidson is No. 15 on pages 252–53 of his book. His discussion of the responses is on pages 49–50. The footnote on page 50 refers specifically to the relationship between his own findings and Coser's. Freidson is careful to point out that his failure to confirm Coser's typology, as a phenomenon independent of social class, should not be taken as conclusive. He suggests further study.

[2] I wish I could say that these similarities were coincidental and, therefore, mutually supportive observations from two different sources. Freidson's work was, of course, familiar to me, though it was not in the forefront of my thinking, when I wrote Chapter One.

[3] Freidson's detailed description of personal interest and competence is on pages 50–56 of his book. I have given a summary which, I hope, is reasonably faithful to the original.

[4] The question asked is No. 24 on page 173 of Feldman (1966), and the findings are described on pages 84–87.

⁵ The discussion on satisfaction and its correlates is on pages 65–75 of Sussman et al. (1967).

⁶ The discussions of the attributes of the good clinic and the good doctor are on pages 241–42 of Fisher (1971). The list of 15 attributes of the good clinic that was submitted to respondents is given on page 241.

⁷ The basic reference to the critical incident technique cited by Sanazaro and Williamson is J.C. Flanagan, "The Critical Incident Technique," *Psychological Bulletin* 5 (1954):327–58. They also cite several applications of the technique to medical care studies. Among these are R.F. Wagner, "A Study of the Critical Requirements for Dentists," *University of Pittsburgh Bulletin* 46 (1950):331–39, and J.T. Bailey, "The Critical Incident Technique in Identifying Behavioral Criteria of a Professional Nursing Effectiveness," *Nursing Research* 5 (1956):52–64.

⁸ Initially a sample of internists' responses was analyzed (Sanazaro and Williamson 1968a, 1968b). Later, responses of surgeons, pediatricians, and obstetricians and gynecologists were also included (Sanazaro and Williamson 1970). The classifications themselves also underwent some small modifications. They appear in final form in Sanazaro and Williamson (1970).

⁹ The table also ignores the distinction between "patient end results" and "process outcomes" that Sanazaro and Williamson used in this and the previous paper (1968a). Patient end results are events that can occur without antecedent medical care, whereas process outcomes are always dependent on prior care. This feature does not appear in the investigators' final classification (1970) but they continue to consider the distinction to be real and useful (Sanazaro and Williamson 1970, p.303).

¹⁰ The data given by Price et al. lend themselves to further interesting analyses which I was unable to make.

References to Chapter Two

Cartwright, A., *Patients and Their Doctors: A Study of General Practice.* New York: Atherton Press, 1967. 295 pp.

Coser, R.L., "A Home Away from Home." *Social Problems* 4 (1956):3–17.

———, *Life in the Ward.* East Lansing, Mich.: Michigan State University Press, 1962. 182 pp.

Feldman, J.J., *The Dissemination of Health Information.* Chicago: Aldine Publishing Co., 1966. 274 pp.

Fisher, A.W., "Patients' Evaluation of Outpatient Medical Care." *Journal of Medical Education* 46 (1971):238–44.

Freidson, E., *Patients' Views of Medical Practice.* New York: Russell Sage Foundation, 1961. 268 pp.

Hopkins, C.E.; Hetherington, R.W.; and Parsons, E.M.; "Quality of Medical Care: A Factor Analysis Approach Using Medical Records." *Health Services Research* 10 (1975):199–208.

Hulka, B.S.; Zyzanski, S.J.; Cassel, J.C.; and Thompson, S.J.; "Satisfaction with Medical Care in a Low Income Population." *Journal of Chronic Diseases* 24 (1971):661–73.

————; Kupper, L.L.; Daly, M.B.; Cassel, J.C.; and Schoen, F.; "Correlates of Satisfaction and Dissatisfaction with Medical Care: A Community Perspective." *Medical Care* 13 (1975):648–58.

Klein, M.W.; Malone, M.F.; Bennis, W.G.; and Berkowitz, N.H.; "Problems of Measuring Patient Care in the Out-Patient Department." *Journal of Health and Human Behavior* 2 (1961):138–44.

Price, P.B.; Taylor, C.W.; Richards, J.M.; and Jacobsen, T.J.; "Measurement of Physician Performance." *Journal of Medical Education* 39 (1964):203–11.

————; Taylor, C.W.; Nelson, D.E.; Lewis, E.G.; Loughmiller, G.C.; Mathiesen, R.; Murray, S.L.; and Maxwell, J.G.; *Measurement and Predictors of Physician Performance: Two Decades of Intermittently Sustained Research.* Salt Lake City, Utah: Aaron Press, 1971. 164 pp.

Riedel, R.L., and Riedel, D.C., *Practice and Performance: An Assessment of Ambulatory Care.* Ann Arbor, Mich.: Health Administration Press, 1979. 306 pp.

Robert Wood Johnson Foundation, *Special Report,* Number One, 1978. 15 pp.

Sanazaro, P.J., and Williamson, J.W., "A Classification of Physician Performance in Internal Medicine." *Journal of Medical Education* 43 (1968):389–97. [1968a]

————, "End Results of Patient Care: A Provisional Classification Based on Reports by Internists." *Medical Care* 6 (1968):123–30. [1968b]

————, "Physician Performance and Its Effects on Patients: A Classification Based on Reports by Internists, Surgeons, Pediatricians, and Obstetricians." *Medical Care* 8 (1970):299–308.

Shiloh, A., "Equalitarian and Hierarchal Patients: An Investigation Among Hadassah Hospital Patients." *Medical Care* 3 (1965):87–95.

Smith, D.B., and Metzner, C.A., "Differential Perceptions of Health Care Quality in a Prepaid Group." *Medical Care* 4 (1970):264–75.

Sussman, M.B.; Caplan, E.K.; Haug, M.R.; and Stern, M.R.; *The Walking Patient: A Study of Outpatient Care.* Cleveland: The Press of the Case Western Reserve University, 1967. 260 pp.

Ware, J.E., and Snyder, M.K., "Dimensions of Patient Attitudes Regarding Doctors and Medical Care Services." *Medical Care* 13 (1975):669–82.

Zyzanski, S.J.; Hulka, B.S.; and Cassel, J.C.; "Scale for the Measurement of 'Satisfaction' with Medical Care: Modifications in Content, Format and Scoring." *Medical Care* 12 (1974):611–20.

THREE

Basic Approaches to
Assessment: Structure,
Process, and Outcome

THREE

The conceptual and empirical explorations of the rather general definition of quality that I have undertaken in the preceding two chapters are
only the first small steps in the analysis of this exasperatingly complex
subject. In this chapter, and in subsequent volumes of the larger work, as
the more general definitions gradually evolve into strategies, criteria, and
standards of measurement, the definition of quality will acquire some
new meanings and will gradually become more concrete and more specific. This does not mean that the final, specific operational measure is
the truest expression of what quality is: I hope that we shall always
return to first principles as we assess the measures themselves. This
should be true also in this chapter, where I consider the basic approaches
or strategies that begin the progression from general principles to more
specific measures.

Structure, Process, and Outcome

I began this book with a definition of quality that embodied an important choice which will now become apparent. By asserting that the
quality of medical care is an attribute that care may have to a greater or a
lesser degree, I have implied that the primary object of study is a set of
activities that go on within and between practitioners and patients. This
set of activities I have called the "process" of care. A judgment concerning
the quality of that process may be made either by direct observation or
by review of recorded information, which allows a more or less accurate
reconstruction of what goes on. But, while "process" is the primary *object*
of assessment, the *basis* for the judgment of quality is what is known
about the relationship between the characteristics of the medical care

process and their consequences to the health and welfare of individuals and of society, in accordance with the value placed upon health and welfare by the individual and by society.

With regard to technical management, the relationship between the characteristics of the process of care and its consequences is determined, in the abstract, by the state of medical science and technology at any given time. More specifically, this relationship is revealed in the work of the leading exponents of that science and technology; through their published research, their teachings, and their own practice these leaders define, explicitly or implicitly, the technical norms of good care.

Another set of norms governs the management of the interpersonal process. These norms arise from the values and the ethical principles and rules that govern the relationships among people, in general, and between health professionals and clients, in particular. By their very nature these norms are postulated as good in themselves; but they can also be seen, on the whole, to contribute to individual and collective welfare.

It follows, therefore, that the quality of the "process" of care is defined, in the first place, as normative behavior. The norms derive either from the science of medicine or from the ethics and values of society. In either case, the norms are meaningful because they contribute to valued consequences. Where social values and ethics are concerned, however, it is important to remember that the norms can be valid independently of their contribution to the more obvious outcomes of care. In fact, in some cases, the preservation of a certain value — for example, the autonomy of the client — may be detrimental to the client, in the judgment of others. Nevertheless, the norm is respected in the service of a broader interest, or a higher principle.

The definition of quality as normative behavior is congenial to the health professions, established as it is by tradition, and almost hallowed by usage. The good physician is required only to do what is known or believed to be best for the patient, leaving the consequences in the hands of the gods, or of the one true God. In more modern times, enlightened by scientific and social "progress," Lee and Jones have embodied this tradition in the following, now classic, definition:

> Good medical care is the kind of medicine practiced and taught by the recognized leaders of the medical profession at a given time or period of social, cultural, and professional development in a community or population group. . . . The concept of good medical care that has been employed in this study is based upon certain "articles of faith" which can be briefly stated.
>
> 1. Good medical care is limited to the practice of rational medicine based on the medical sciences.
>
> · · ·

2. Good medical care emphasizes prevention.

    . . .

3. Good medical care requires intelligent cooperation between the lay public and the practitioners of scientific medicine.

    . . .

4. Good medical care treats the individual as a whole.

    . . .

5. Good medical care maintains a close and continuing personal relation between physician and patient.

    . . .

6. Good medical care is coordinated with social welfare work.

    . . .

7. Good medical care coordinates all types of medical services.

    . . .

8. Good medical care implies the application of all the necessary services of modern scientific medicine to the needs of all the people. (Lee and Jones 1933, pp.6–10)[1]

A more detailed specification of the attributes of quality, one that derives from the work of Lee and Jones, is offered the reader in Appendix A.

I have argued, so far, that the most direct route to an assessment of the quality of care is an examination of that care. But there are, in my opinion, two other, less direct approaches to assessment: one of these is the assessment of "structure," and the other the assessment of "outcome."

By "structure" I mean the relatively stable characteristics of the providers of care, of the tools and resources they have at their disposal, and of the physical and organizational settings in which they work. The concept of structure includes the human, physical, and financial resources that are needed to provide medical care. The term embraces the number, distribution, and qualifications of professional personnel, and so, too, the number, size, equipment, and geographic disposition of hospitals and other facilities. But the concept also goes beyond the factors of production to include the ways in which the financing and delivery of health services are organized, both formally and informally. The presence of health insurance is an aspect of structure. So is the manner in which physicians conduct their work, in individual practice or in groups, and so is the way they are paid. Structure includes the organization of the medical or nursing staff in a hospital, and the presence or absence of a quality review effort, as well as its characteristics, in all their detail. The basic characteristics of structure are that it is relatively stable, that it functions to produce care or is a feature of the "environment" of care, and that it influences the kind of care that is provided.

The use of structure as an indirect measure of the quality of care depends on the nature of its influence on care. When they are present, features of structure that are known or believed to have a salutary effect on the quality of care are taken to be indirect evidence of quality. Other features, known or believed to have a deleterious effect, are taken as evidence of poor quality. Structure, therefore, is relevant to quality in that it increases or decreases the probability of good performance. There are, of course, many attributes of structure that may be desirable or undesirable for reasons other than their contribution to the quality of care. These attributes are irrelevant to assessments of the quality of care, though they could be relevant to. another set of considerations used to judge the "quality" of medical care institutions, programs, or systems.

The relationship between structure and the quality of care is, of course, of the greatest importance in the planning, design, and implementation of systems that are intended to provide personal health services. But as a means for assessing the quality of care, structure is a rather blunt instrument; it can only indicate general tendencies. The usefulness of structure as an indicator of the quality of care is also limited because of our insufficient knowledge about the relationships between structure and performance. It remains to be seen what improvements in specificity and sensitivity can be achieved by the development of more detailed, more condition-specific structural requirements, such as those proposed by Blum (1974). Finally, the relative stability of structure makes it unsuitable for continuous monitoring, though it should be subjected to intermittent checking.

I believe that good structure, that is, a sufficiency of resources and proper system design, is probably the most important means of protecting and promoting the quality of care. This should come as no surprise, since good structure incorporates a well-designed mechanism for monitoring the quality of care and for acting on its findings. But this book is about quality assessment and monitoring, and not about how medical care systems should be designed or organized. As a source of accurate current information about quality, the assessment of structure is of a good deal less importance than the assessment of process or outcome. For this reason, and because I must put some limits on my own work, structure will receive little attention in this volume. But in a review of illustrative studies of the quality of care, which I hope to prepare later, I shall take pains to describe what they say about the relationship between structure and performance. Such findings are the groundwork for the more successful use of structure in the assessment of quality, and also for the means to design a system that encourages and rewards good performance.

The study of "outcomes" is the other of the indirect approaches that I have said could be used to assess the quality of care. In this book I shall use "outcome" to mean a change in a patient's current and future health status that can be attributed to antecedent health care. By postulating a rather broad definition of health, I shall include improvement of social and psychological function in addition to the more usual emphasis on the physical and physiological aspects of performance. By still another extension I shall add patient attitudes (including satisfaction), health-related knowledge acquired by the patient, and health-related behavioral change. All of these can be seen either as components of current health or as contributions to future health.

It seems paradoxical to define the quality of care in terms of changes in health status, and yet to regard changes in health status as an indirect measure of the quality of care, rather than as the most direct measure of all. After many years, during which this formulation has been challenged by many scholars for whom I have the highest regard, I have remained faithful to it, partly for a reason that I might call semantic. It seems to me that when we speak of the quality of care, we are concerned with the most immediately discernible attributes of that care; and these can be most clearly seen as normative behavior. Another reason, one that is more substantive, is that there is nothing that is clearly a more direct measure of the quality of care. Obviously, "structure" does not qualify. As to changes in health status, they do not serve as a measure of the quality of care until other causes for such changes have been eliminated, and one is reasonably sure that previous care is responsible for the change, which then can be truly called an "outcome." One can, of course, turn this coin over and say, with at least equal force, that elements of the process of care do not signify quality until their relationship to desirable changes in health status has been established. In a general sense this is true. But, once it has been established that certain procedures used in specified situations are clearly associated with good results, the mere presence or absence of these procedures in these situations can be accepted as evidence of good or bad quality. There is no need for further ascertainment. I do not believe that changes in health status offer an analogous situation. When changes in health status are observed, there must not only be a prior basis for assuming a possible relationship to antecedent care; further ascertainment is also often needed, at least to show the absence of other factors that might explain the findings, preferably together with the presence of the kind of care that can explain them.

I shall return to the duality, real or imagined, of process and outcome as a means for assessing the quality of care. For now, all that is needed is to accept, provisionally, that there are three major approaches to quality assessment: "structure," "process," and "outcome." This three-fold approach is possible because there is a fundamental functional relationship among the three elements, which can be shown schematically as follows:

Structure → Process → Outcome.

This means that structural characteristics of the settings in which care takes place have a propensity to influence the process of care so that its quality is diminished or enhanced. Similarly, changes in the process of care, including variations in its quality, will influence the effect of care on health status, broadly defined. And given this way of thinking, it becomes easier to generate and classify a variety of more specific indicators of quality, such as those I have shown in Appendix B.

Although this formulation rests on certain basic relationships that are of great theoretical and operational significance, it is offered here mainly as a useful way of organizing one's thinking about the rather confused field of quality assessment and monitoring. To that end, I have tried to define the three components of the triad as carefully as I can. But I know that many ambiguities remain, as becomes apparent when one tries to classify specific phenomena exclusively under one of the three headings. This is because the three-part division is a somewhat arbitrary abstraction from what is, in reality, a succession of less clearly differentiated, but causally related, elements in a chain that probably has many branches. In such a chain, each element is, at least to some extent, a cause of the element that follows, while it is itself caused by the elements that precede it. In an insightful analysis, Simon has pointed out that in a chain of this kind it is futile to try to distinguish means from ends. The analyst's purposes and perspectives determine what segment of the chain he will study, and what is a means and what is an end (Simon 1961). For example, by placing "outcomes" at the end of my three-part progression I have assumed that the amelioration of "health" is the primary objective of medical care.[2] But, in another context, health could be a means to another end: for example, economic development. In still another situation, it may be appropriate to stop short of changes in health status in specifying the objectives of a medical care system. Alternatively, the process of care may be subdivided into smaller segments, each with its own "outcome." Here are some examples.

In an early study that is an important step in the history of quality assessment, Makover saw "the end product of medical care" to be "the actual medical service rendered." (Makover 1951, p.825) Makover's formulation had only two components which were, according to my terminology, (1) structure, represented by the policies, organization, administration, and finances of the prepaid groups which he studied, and (2) process, which was the care produced, and which Makover took to be the "end product" of these groups.

Makover's formulation antedates mine, so that I have had to reinterpret his viewpoint in the light of subsequent developments. A more recent proposal by Doll openly rejects the trinitarian view of quality assessment in favor of another form of dualism which, this time, excludes structure, but affirms process and outcome! In his words, "I have not separated structure, despite common usage, as it seems to me a part of the process by which outcome is affected." (Doll 1974, p.305)

In another deliberate reformulation, Williamson has introduced a system of assessment which begins with certain outcomes and works backward to the processes that led to them (Williamson 1971). If this sequence is reversed, Williamson's formulation can be superimposed on mine in the following progression:

$$\text{structure} \rightarrow \frac{\text{diagnostic}}{\text{process}} \rightarrow \frac{\text{diagnostic}}{\text{outcome}} \rightarrow \frac{\text{therapeutic}}{\text{process}} \rightarrow \frac{\text{therapeutic}}{\text{outcomes.}}$$

What Williamson has done is to divide the category of process into two segments, representing diagnostic and therapeutic activities. The outcomes of therapy (and all that precedes it) are perceived as a change in health status. The outcome of diagnostic activity is, in an immediate sense, a diagnosis. But this, usually, represents a completed step in a progression rather than an end in itself. In an earlier publication I suggested that elements such as this be called "procedural endpoints" rather than outcomes (Donabedian 1966, p.169). Since this suggestion has been ignored, I must asume that there is something inappropriate or unattractive about it.

The examples I have cited show that the tripartite division into structure, process, and outcome is open to a variety of modifications. I believe that these modifications are both legitimate and helpful, as long as they are correctly understood and properly used. In that spirit I would like to review some important alternative formulations and to comment on their similarities, their differences, and their implications.

Alternative Formulations

The trilogy of process, structure, and outcome has both antecedents and descendents. Among the antecedents the most important is to be found in a paper by Mindel Sheps that has deeply influenced my thinking (Sheps 1955). In it Sheps maps out, perhaps for the first time, the broad domain of quality assessment, introducing order where previously confusion had prevailed. According to Sheps, "The main technique used in appraisals of hospital quality can be divided into:

The examination of prerequisites or desiderata for adequate care.

Indexes of elements of performance.

Indexes of the effects of care.

Qualitative clinical evaluations." (Sheps 1955, p.879)

In pondering this classification and the descriptions of its elements, I came to see that with a small rearrangement three elements would emerge, and that these could be well described as structure, process, and outcome. The first two segments of Table 3-1 show the correspondence

TABLE 3-1

ALTERNATIVE FORMULATIONS OF APPROACHES TO
QUALITY ASSESSMENT AND PROGRAM EVALUATION
AND THEIR INTERRELATIONSHIPS.

Investigator   *Elements of the Formulation*

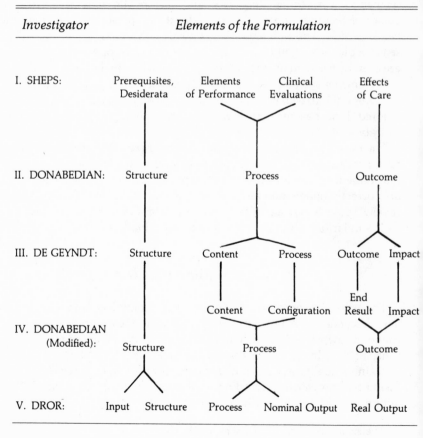

Sources: Sheps 1955; Donabedian 1966; De Geyndt 1970; Dror 1968.

Among the formulations that followed mine, one of the most interesting was proposed by De Geyndt in 1970. It is an instructive reformulation not only because it offers an alternative to the basic trilogy, but also because it illustrates very clearly the influence on the formulation of what I have called the level and scope of concern.[3] If I understand De Geyndt correctly, a major element in his model is the inclusivity of the definition of health, and the span of the gamut of health services that corresponds to that definition. At the narrowest, these services are confined to the care of illness. At their broadest, they comprise, in a rough progression, the promotion of social and mental health, the promotion of physical health, preventive supervision, the prevention of illness, early diagnosis, care of illness, physical rehabilitation, and social rehabilitation. The set of activities and the criteria that enter the definition and assessment of quality correspond to which of the elements of this progression are legitimately included or excluded.

De Geyndt also emphasizes the importance of the difference between analysis at the level of individuals and analysis at the level of communities or populations, as well as that of the differences that are introduced when attention shifts from episodes of care to longer sequences. The first of these distinctions leads him to distinguish "outcomes," which are primarily changes in physical health in individuals, from "impact," which is the effect of the broader gamut of health services on the entire population, under a more inclusive definition of health. Thus, De Geyndt's distinction between "outcome" and "impact" seems to be based partly on the level of analysis (individual versus aggregate) and partly on the inclusivity of the definition of health (physical-physiological versus something akin to the quality of life).

The second distinction, that between episodic care and sequences of care, leads De Geyndt to make a corresponding distinction between the discrete activities that go into care, which he calls "content," and the organization of these activities, which he calls "process." This latter category includes the attributes of continuity, coordination, teamwork, and appropriate sequencing.

One result of these considerations is the break-up of the structure-process-outcome trilogy into the more closely detailed quasi-sequence of "structure," "content," "process," "outcome" and "impact." It seems to me, however, that both the general model and the more specific categories proposed by De Geyndt are closely congruent with mine. The second and third rows of Table 3-1 show one aspect of that correspondence;[4] and in the fourth row I have proposed a nomenclature that reconciles the two formulations, while it avoids the use of the same words to mean somewhat different things.

The correspondence between De Geyndt's formulation and mine suggests a certain plausibility and usefulness, if not validity, in the general approach that both formulations represent. Additional support comes from an entirely different field. In a work on the assessment of public policy, Yehezkel Dror has proposed a sequence, which is represented in the fifth row of Table 3-1 (Dror 1968). In Dror's formulation, "input" includes (1) qualified manpower and their time, (2) knowledge which is additional to that inherent in the qualifications of the manpower, (3) equipment, including that used in information processing, and (4) energy and drive. Dror recognizes the input of money as an important consideration, but argues that, in the process of evaluation, money inputs will have to be translated into their more specific representations. The mix or balance of inputs could perhaps be seen as an additional category, since, in Dror's words, "the way the various inputs are mixed lends them a significance much greater than the sum of their individual significances." (Dror 1968, p.57) It is a small step from here to "structure," which is the way in which the inputs are organized in the formulation and execution of public policy. As to the "process" of policy formulation, it is seen to have two consequences. The first of these is the policy itself. In Dror's formulation, this is called the "nominal output." A plan for patient management, including investigation and treatment, would correspond, I believe, to Dror's "nominal output." If this is so, this could be considered a "procedural end point," according to my terminology. The "real output," in Dror's formulation, is the actual effect of the policy, which corresponds to the categories of outcome, end result, or impact, as they are used in models of quality assessment.

The work of Williamson occupies a special position among these alternative formulations. I have already described how Williamson, earlier in the course of his work, divided the process of care into its diagnostic and therapeutic components, identifying a diagnosis as the outcome of the first, and a change in health as the outcome of the second. In Williamson's later work, the concept of outcome is still further broadened to encompass "any characteristic of patients, health problems, providers, or their interaction in the care process that results from care provided or required, as measured at one point in time." (Williamson 1978, p.26) In a formulation that is reminiscent of Simon's means-ends chain, Williamson sees the process of care as a succession of causally linked events. This flow, which Williamson likens to that of a motion picture, constitutes "process." But, as when a film is stopped, each element in this previously unfolding succession, when isolated for scrutiny, is really an outcome, provided that it is causally related to antecedent states and events about which a judgment is to be made. And, in fact, so is the entire train of events, when we examine them in their static form, as if they have been frozen in time. Thus, the history that is taken, the physical examination that is performed, and the laboratory tests that are ordered are all outcomes of subparts of the diagnostic process, just as the final diagnostic designation is an outcome of this process as a whole. Similarly, the performance of surgery and the institution of drug treatment are two outcomes that are found in the course of the therapeutic process, the more nearly final outcome of which is some amelioration in health status, physical, psychological, or social. In this new light, the traditional methods of utilization review, chart audit, and profile analysis, as these are widely practiced, are seen by Williamson as forms of outcome assessment (p.28). By contrast, the measurement of process "requires direct observation over time," for example, by "audiovisual means," so that one may judge whether the procedures that constitute care are themselves "validly and adequately accomplished." (Williamson 1978, pp.34, 35)

I would conclude from this exposition that the mere performance of any element of care is a criterion of outcome, as long as it is causally linked to some prior activity. To convert this into the "process" category would require direct observation of how well that element of care is performed. It is hard to say what else might be included under this concept of process. For Williamson, having drained the concept of almost all of its traditional content, seems to have no interest in what remains. But, should one include the more dynamic attributes of timing, sequence, continuity, coordination, and the like, one would restore to process some of its lost dignity, ending up with a concept not unlike that proposed by De Geyndt (1970). In this way, Williamson's more radical formulation, which seemed to threaten to all but destroy the distinctions that are usually made between process and outcome, may yet be accommodated within the bounds of the more traditional framework.

In my opinion, the basic formulation of structure, process, and outcome gains in validity and usefulness as a result of all these comparisons. Its validity is strengthened by its overt or latent presence as a substrate in these other formulations. Its usefulness is enhanced by its demonstrated flexibility, since it lends itself to considerable adaptation and elaboration, without the loss of its fundamental classificatory or conceptual significance. From the beginning, I have offered "structure," "process," and "outcome" as a guide, not a straightjacket. The reader should feel free to select from the formulations I have shown in Table 3-1 any that seem appropriate to his needs, to develop a formulation that combines elements of several, or to create a new formulation of his own. For example, the ecumenical formulation that appeals to me the most would be something like what follows:

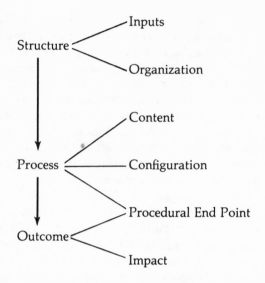

But, tomorrow, I could change my mind: and I would advise the reader, in the colorful argot of our day, to hang equally loose, provided that he has an unshakable grasp of the fundamentals!

I have also, from the very beginning, offered "structure," "process," and "outcome" not as attributes of quality, but as approaches to the acquisition of information about the presence or absence of the attributes that constitute or define quality. An explicit application of this principle is found in a scheme for assessing and monitoring the effectiveness of health policy and practice that was proposed by Doll in 1974. According to Doll, "This field has three aspects — medical efficacy, social accept-ability and economic efficiency — that are independent of one another and require different methods of evaluation. Moreover each aspect can be monitored in terms of the outcome achieved or the process by which the outcome is reached." (Doll 1974, p.305) I have already commented on Doll's decision to include structure as part of process in his formula-tion. Another feature worthy of remark is Doll's emphasis on the sepa-rateness of the three "aspects" of effectiveness. This differs from the emphasis in my "unified model," in which I try to join the three aspects, to the greatest extent possible. But what I want to dwell on now is not these differences, but the similarities between our points of view, which result in the cross-tabulation of the three attributes of effectiveness and the two approaches to assessment, to form the matrix shown in Table 3-2. There is no doubt that a matrix of this kind is a useful tool for classi-fying methods of assessment, and perhaps for finding some that do not immediately come to mind. Unfortunately (for our purposes, but not necessarily for his), Professor Doll does not go on to use the matrix in this way. He decides, for good reasons, to "give most attention to outcome"; and in the instances where he may have used measures of structure or process he does not explicitly say so. As a result, I have had to use my own judgment to classify some of the measures that Doll has proposed, and to add a few others in order to fill the matrix. But this should not distract the reader, since the matrix shown in Table 3-2 is meant only to be illustrative of the way in which the cross-tabulation of attributes and approaches can map out a complicated domain.

Another similar example can be found in the work of Freeborn and Greenlick, who have proposed a comprehensive classification of approaches to assessing the performance of ambulatory care systems (Freeborn and Greenlick 1973). This classification is shown in abridged form in Table 3-3, and in greater detail in Appendix C. Here I shall examine only its major characteristics, and relate these to the dominant themes of this chapter. In doing so I hope to show that the classification proposed by Freeborn and Greenlick grows out of, or can be reconciled with, the perspectives and formulations that I have already described, provided that allowances are made for the fact that their classification deals with the assessment of the patient-physician interaction as part of the evaluation of an entire program of personal health care.[5]

Reference to Table 3-3 will show that, according to Freeborn and Greenlick, there are two major subdivisions to program evaluation: the assessment of effectiveness and the assessment of efficiency. The first subdivision is, in its turn, divided into two large categories: technical effectiveness and psychosocial effectiveness. The methods for assessing technical effectiveness are classified under the now-familiar headings of structure, process, and outcome; and the process of care includes, as would be congenial to De Geyndt, not only the activities of the providers, but the attributes of accessibility and continuity as well. But, from here on, structure, process, and outcome are not used as organizing categories. Instead, the studies of psychosocial effectiveness are divided into those that are aimed at either patient or provider satisfaction; and each of these may deal either with attitudes (such as satisfaction) or with behaviors (such as leaving the ambulatory care plan).

To simplify matters, I shall not discuss the assessment of efficiency. As to effectiveness, it seems to me that the categories of structure, process, and outcome suffice to organize psychosocial effectiveness just as well as they organize technical effectiveness. As I see it, the classification proposed by Freeborn and Greenlick looks into three attributes of "technical effectiveness" which are listed in something of a temporal sequence as "accessibility," "provider performance," and "continuity." One can also

TABLE 3-2

A Matrix for Assessing and Monitoring the Effectiveness of Health Policy and Practice, Based on a Proposal by Doll, 1974.

Attributes That Define or Constitute Effectiveness	Approaches to Assessment and Monitoring	
	Process (including structure)	*Outcome*
Medical Efficacy	1. Use of service relative to need, as revealed by morbidity surveys (2. Adherence to professionally defined criteria and standards of care)	1. Mortality by age group and by locality 2. Disease-specific mortality 3. Fatality by provider category, by hospital, etc. 4. Morbidity: existing data and special surveys 5. Indexes of health and performance
Social Acceptability	1. Waiting time for appointments, hospital admissions, etc. 2. Equal opportunity for equal treatment for patients at equal risk; roughly indicated by allocation of funds	1. Public satisfaction or dissatisfaction inferred from complaints, political pressures, etc. 2. Surveys of public opinion (3. Equalization of health status among social groups, localities, etc.)
Economic Efficiency	1. Differences in hospital lengths of stay; changes over time (2. Size of facilities relative to function) (3. Appropriateness of allocation of functions to classes of personnel)	1. Health effects of early mobilization and discharge from hospital 2. Cost of achieving specified improvements in health as shown by cost-benefit analysis

Source: Based on Doll 1974. I have used my own judgment in summarizing and classifying a selection of the measures that Doll proposed and evaluated. I have also added some measures that Doll did not mention. These are shown in parentheses.

TABLE 3-3

Major Categories in a Classification of
Approaches to the Assessment of the Performance
of Ambulatory Care Systems, as Proposed by
Freeborn and Greenlick, 1973.

I. Assessment of Effectiveness

A. Technical Effectiveness

1. Structure
2. Process of providing care

a. Accessibility
b. Provider performance
c. Continuity

3. Technical outcome of care

B. Psychosocial Effectiveness

1. Patient satisfaction

a. Attitudinal measures
b. Behavioral observations

2. Provider satisfaction

a. Attitudinal measures
b. Behavioral observations

II. Assessment of Efficiency

A. Relation between input and output
B. Relation between cost and output

Source: Abridged from Freeborn and Greenlick 1973.

infer that "provider performance" is perceived as divisible into the two areas that correspond to what I have called technical management and the management of the interpersonal process. Partly explicit and partly implicit is the postulate that each of these attributes can be assessed by examining structure, process, and outcome. Freeborn and Greenlick, however, at least implicitly, subdivide the three major approaches into five classes. For example, it is possible to infer a division of structure into the physical and the socioorganizational. The category of process includes not only activities but also procedural end points, such as making a diagnosis. But the most significant departure from earlier formulations is in the category of outcomes. By including "provider satisfaction," in addition to "patient satisfaction," as a measure of system effectiveness, Freeborn and Greenlick open the way to a distinction between client-related and practitioner-related outcomes, though they do not present their classification in this way, nor use these terms. They do, however, make a very useful distinction between the study of attitudes and the study of behaviors as alternative ways of learning about the satisfaction of patients and providers. They also mention a variety of what I would call "client-related outcomes" that could be classified as follows:

1. Cognitive: knowledge on the part of the patient about his current health problem and its management; knowledge about health problems in general; knowledge about how to go about receiving care, in the particular situation and in general.
2. Attitudinal: feelings and attitudes about the items mentioned under the cognitive category. Judgments about the settings, the process, and the outcome of care, in a specific situation and in general.
3. Behavioral:
   a. Use of health services in the specific situation and in general, including timely seeking of care, volume of care, adherence to the regimen of care, the sources of care, and the stability of the patient-practitioner relationship.
   b. Health promotion relevant to the specific health problem and in general, including changes in diet, activity, and rest, in use of cigarettes and drugs, and so on.
   c. Health status, including mobility, morbidity, disability, and performance in the physical-physiological, emotional-psychological, and social realms.

It is possible to use this interpretation to recast the classification offered by Freeborn and Greenlick into a matrix similar to that shown in Table 3-2. But this would be so awkward to reproduce that I will present it, instead, in the form of a list, using mainly items I have drawn from the Freeborn and Greenlick classification, but adding some other items as well. By doing so I am, emphatically, *not* saying that the alternative formulation is any better than, or even as good as, the original. I simply want to demonstrate, once again, the way in which the cross-tabulation of attributes and approaches was intended to classify the methods and measures of assessment. And I am doing this once more, using a more complicated classification, because I hope it will strengthen the reader's grasp of the matter. Having laid down this groundwork, we can now go to the classification itself.

A. Accessibility: Physical and Socioorganizational
1. Structure
Geographic factors such as distance, isolation, and geographic availability and accessibility of services and facilities. The presence of well-defined and well-known points of entry to care. Scope and nature of benefits and services. System arrangements, including provision for drop-ins, emergencies, coverage at night and on weekends, and home visits. Population characteristics (demographic, social, economic, locational) that are relevant to the preceding features.
2. Process
Timeliness and delay in seeking care.[6] Utilization patterns by time, place, type of illness or reason for seeking care, and type of provider, especially when related to need and to sociodemographic and residential characteristics of the clients. Adherence of personnel to clinic hours; absenteeism.
3. Client-related Outcomes
Undiagnosed disease, preventable disease, morbidity, mortality, disability. Satisfaction with accessibility; use of service outside the plan. Social, demographic, and residential differences in the preceding measures which would suggest differences in accessibility to care.
4. Practitioner-related Outcomes
Satisfaction with, and opinions about, accessibility and the arrangements made to enhance it. Dissatisfaction with excessive accessibility.
B. Technical Management
1. Structure
Physical structure, facilities, and equipment. Range and scope of services. Ownership, accreditation, and affiliation status of hospitals and other facilities. Numbers, types, and qualifications of staff. Staff organization. Fiscal organization, including financing and methods of payment. The presence and organization of quality-monitoring mechanisms. Satisfaction of practitioners and other staff with the conditions of work, including facilities, equipment, staffing, remuneration, relationships with colleagues, relationships with patients, prestige, opportunities for learning, etc.
2. Process
Characteristics of use of service relative to need. Adequacy of diagnostic work-up and treatment, including the completeness and specificity of the diagnosis. Adherence to professionally defined

norms of good practice, both in general and for specific conditions, diagnoses, and situations.
3. Client-related Outcomes
Mortality and disability, in general and in special subgroups. Occurrence of undetected or preventable morbidity and disability. Results of treatment in the form of complications, fatality, residual disability, or the restoration of physical, psychological, and social function. Client satisfaction with the outcomes as well as the structural characteristics and the process that are perceived to lead to the outcomes.
4. Practitioner-related Outcomes
Satisfaction with equipment, facilities, qualifications of colleagues, and opportunity for consultation. Satisfaction with time allowed for patient care, and with conditions suitable for doing good work without administrative interference. Satisfaction with type and degree of supervision. Opinions about the quality of care. Resignations attributed to dissatisfaction concerning conditions necessary to provide good care.
C. The Management of the Interpersonal Process
1. Structure
Stability of attachment to a personal physician. Availability of adequate time for physicians to spend with patients.[7] The amenities incorporated in the physical setup and the operations of the facility. The presence and the functioning of adequate mechanisms for dealing with client suggestions and complaints. Consumer participation in governance. Satisfaction of practitioners and other personnel with the conditions of work and with its material and psychic rewards.
2. Process
The manner in which practitioners and other personnel deal with patients. Concern, courtesy, respect for the client's autonomy, maintaining privacy, explanation, reassurance, support; nonjudgmental acceptance of the patient, his illness, and his behavior. Use of enough time; not rushing the patient.
3. Client-related Outcomes
Satisfaction with the amenities of care and aspects of the interpersonal relationship. Understanding of illness and regimen of care. Adherence to regimen. Change of primary practitioners within the plan. Use of services outside the plan. In general, establishment of behaviors that indicate successful coping with illness and disability, improvements in prospects for future health, and greater ability to seek and to use care appropriately.

4. Practitioner-related Outcomes
Satisfaction with relationships with clients. Opinions about patient behaviors. Knowledge of client concerns and problems.[8]
D. Continuity
1. Structure
Arrangements to assure a central, coordinated source of care, such as a primary physician. Arrangements for referrals and for follow-up. Arrangements for maintaining and retrieving information that contributes to coherent and consistent management.[9] Staff turnover and average length of time in position.
2. Process
Number of physicians and facilities involved in the care received by the client, with and without referral.[10] Interruptions of relationships with personal physician, frequency of unscheduled visits, use of outside physicians without referral. Frequency and appropriateness of referral. Degree of follow-up on abnormal findings. Follow-up on broken appointments. Checks on adherence to regimen. Evidence of use of past information in current management.[11]
3. Client-related Outcomes
Adherence to prescribed regimen. Broken appointments. Use of outside physicians without referral. Untoward consequences to health status. Client satisfaction with arrangements for continuity, and the resulting stability of the patient-practitioner relationship. Client's ability to identify the primary source of care.[12]
4. Practitioner-related Outcomes
Satisfaction with arrangements and procedures to ensure continuity. Knowledge of patient's past medical and social history, the home situation, environmental stresses and hazards, patient concerns, coping abilities and weakness, etc.

A study of this classification, which is mainly a rearrangement of the one proposed by Freeborn and Greenlick, shows that, by and large, it works, even though we might disagree in some instances as to precisely where certain items belong — especially as to whether something belongs more appropriately under process or under outcome. But, in addition to providing convenient boxes in which to store what may be an over-abundance of items, the classification seems also to work as a device that triggers new departures in a search for, or a rediscovery of, additional methods and measures of assessment. What is perhaps most important of all, the use of the classification is likely to reveal conceptual and functional relationships which, once discovered, may seem to have been obvious all along. One such relationship is the tendency of the same kinds of outcomes to appear in many positions of the classification. This is because certain outcomes — for example, changes in health status — have an integrative property, in that they represent the final, joint effects of many factors that influence clinical performance. In this particular case, it also became clear to me, for the first time, that certain outcomes, particularly those that are practitioner-related, can become part of structure. Among these are the orientations, behaviors, and satisfactions or dissatisfactions of those who provide care. By becoming part of the environment in which care is provided, from that point on these features influence the quality of care and the effectiveness of the system. Established biases in the thinking and behavior of clients may play a similar role.

The classification proposed by Doll came ready-made for my purposes. The classification described by Freeborn and Greenlick is so congenial to my thinking that it was easy to twist it into the shape I wanted, much as a circus clown deftly makes a pretzel from what seems to be an iron rod, simply because the rod is actually made of rubber. I shall now try something a little harder, since it involves a classification that was developed with the avowed purpose of joining, rather than separating, the categories of structure, process, and outcome.

Not too long ago, Lane and Kelman set out to construct a conceptual framework for evaluating the quality of maternal health care that would be comprehensive, that "links structure, process and outcome variables," and that is applicable to "a population of expectant mothers and their infants in a community, not the care rendered by a single program, or physician, or hospital." (Lane and Kelman 1975, pp.804, 799) The classification, which is reproduced in Appendix D, begins with two basic elements: (1) "system functional characteristics," and (2) "system objectives." The "functional characteristics" of the system are conceived to be "accessibility, availability, adequacy, responsiveness and effectiveness." The objectives of the system are visualized as prevention, minimization of adverse consequences, maintenance of health, and rehabilitation. Lists of "indicators" are then developed for each of these categories, with the indicators further classified according to whether they are pertinent to (1) the prenatal period, (2) labor and delivery, or (3) postpartum care. There are, altogether, 322 "indicators" of quality, in nine lists, each with three subparts. In addition, the investigators indicate the source of information for each indicator.

As shown in Table 3-4, even this massive accumulation of material can be rather neatly arranged in a matrix that cross-tabulates attributes and approaches. The only important change I have made in the framework proposed by Lane and Kelman is the classification of "effectiveness" as a separate category from the others, on the ground that it is the only one that deals with outcomes — which, in their turn, represent the net effect of many of the other characteristics of the system, and of the care it produces. As the Table shows very clearly, system attributes related to accessibility, availability, and responsiveness are measured almost exclusively by "indicators" that describe structure. Adequacy, the fourth attribute of the system, is defined as "the extent to which needed, or indicated, services are sufficient quantitatively or qualitatively." (Lane and Kelman 1975, p.796) Perhaps as a result of this melding of quantity and quality, indicators both of structure and of process are used to measure adequacy, as is shown in Table 3-4. Only descriptions of process are provided as indicators for prevention, minimization of adverse conse-

TABLE 3-4

A Matrix Showing the Positions Occupied by
the Categories of Indicators of the Quality of
Maternal Health Care Proposed by Lane and
Kelman, 1975.

Categories Proposed by Lane and Kelman		Approaches to Assessment		
		Structure	Process	Outcome
System Attributes:	Accessibility	X		
	Availability	X		
	Responsiveness	X		
	Adequacy	X	X	
Care Characteristics:	Prevention		X	
	Minimization*		X	
	Maintenance†		X	
	Rehabilitation		X	
Effectiveness				X

Source: Based on Lane and Kelman 1975.
*Minimization of adverse consequences.
†Maintenance of health.
The X marks indicate the location of each of the indicators proposed by Lane and Kelman.

quences, health maintenance, and rehabilitation. For this reason, I have
called these categories characteristics of care rather than system objectives, as it was originally proposed. Effectiveness is indicated entirely by
outcomes, provided outcomes are taken to include not only changes in
health status, but also client satisfaction, knowledge, and health-related
behavior. But perhaps the blank spaces are as important as what is included in the matrix. These conspicuous absences show that a host of
indicators, as yet unconceived, are waiting to be born.[13]

The Choice of an Approach: Process or Outcome?

The title for this section poses a choice between process and outcome
partly for dramatic effect, but mainly because this is the way in which the
choice is usually presented in the often polemical literature of recent
years. But we should remember that when information about process
and outcome is not available, an examination of structure is the only
remaining method for assessment or monitoring; and that structure con-
tinues to be an important supplement when information about process
and outcome is available but incomplete. Also, as I have already said,
structure, by which I mean adequate resources and proper program design, is perhaps the most important single factor in what most people
now call "quality assurance" (even though this is, I think, too optimistic a
term). The monitoring function, whether external or internal to the
organization, is, itself, a part of the structure. Moreover, other aspects of
structure influence the effective performance of monitoring; and many
aspects of structure — including, but also going much beyond, the monitoring function — can have an important effect on the behavior of practitioners and of clients. Thus, the prior specification of program design,
and periodic checks to make sure that the specifications are still in force,
is an important method for assessing the propensity of an organization to
encourage or discourage "good" performance. This means that even
though structure may have a subsidiary role in the assessing and monitoring of actual performance, it is fundamental to an assessment of the
potential, capacity, or propensity to perform badly or well.

Having paid due respect to structure, we can now turn to the two main
contenders in the ring. I choose this metaphor advisedly, since the situation is often presented as if it were a contest in which there can be only
one winner. I think this view of the situation is a false one, or, at least, it
is overly simplified. But I must also admit that there seems to be a curious
dualism that attracts people to either one or the other of the two camps —
the one that has pledged allegiance to process, or the other that accepts

no master other than outcome. It is my impression that the more traditional clinicians are to be found in the first group, whereas the second
group harbors the nihilists and the iconoclasts who either delight in, or
are weighed down by, what they believe to be the uselessness of a great
deal of what constitutes contemporary medicine. Also to be found in the
second camp are many health planners, policy makers, and administrators, who fear that the emphasis on process will increase costs without
producing corresponding improvements in health. And, finally, there are
those who have turned to outcomes because they have been disappointed
by the imprecision and the costliness of the assessments of process.

Between these two camps, the balance of influence has tilted, in recent
years, in favor of outcomes. It is now a badge of honor, an assurance of
almost immediate acceptance, to say that a method of assessment is based
on outcome. Conversely, a method that is said to be based on process is
greeted with skepticism, if not outright contempt. No wonder, then, that
methods of assessment are presented in a manner that will emphasize
their use of outcomes, while it will play down or conceal components
that depend on the assessment of process.[14]

Partisanship such as this may add color and excitement to life in the
world of action, and to engage in it would perhaps liven up even these
tedious pages. But it is wiser to resist the temptation, and to look, instead, at a basic set of issues which bear on the selection and use of any
approach to assessment.

Validity

The relative validity of each of the two rival approaches is the most
important point at issue in the arguments of their detractors and sup-
porters. But the concept of validity is itself made up of many parts; and
there is no precise way of saying what belongs to it, or what belongs
more appropriately under another heading. With the hope that the reader
will allow me some flexibility of classification, I would say that the question of validity covers two large domains. The first has to do with the
accuracy of the data and the precision of the measures that are constructed with these data. The second has to do with the justifiability of
the inferences that are drawn from the data and the measurements.

I will have more to say about data and measurements in a subsequent
volume of this work. There our concern shall be with, for example, the
veracity and the completeness of the information obtained from medical
records, from other documents and reports, and from clients by direct
questioning. When we look at these matters, we shall find it difficult to
decide which of the two, process or outcome, is the more open to misrep-

resentation as a result of deficiencies in the data. The same can be said about many scales and measures that are constructed for the use of these data. Generalities about validity are likely to fail us; in each instance we shall have to consider the particular phenomenon, the particular source of information, and the particular measure, irrespective of whether we are dealing with an element of process or an element of outcome.

The justifiability of *inferences* about quality does, however, lend itself to some generalization, owing to certain fundamental properties and relationships that distinguish process from outcome. But, even here, it is important to reexamine on its own merits each particular use of each specific measure that leads to any given inference.

Taken by and large, outcomes tend to be inherently valid, in the sense that there is usually no need to argue whether they are, in themselves, good or bad. For example, there is general agreement that life is preferable to death, functional integrity preferable to disability, and comfort preferable to pain. By contrast, the validity of the elements of process is fundamentally derivative, because it depends on the contribution of process to desired outcomes. But there are important exceptions. As I have already said, there are some attributes of the interpersonal process that are valid in themselves, because they represent approved or desirable behaviors in specified social situations. Attributes such as these may be valued and preserved even though they make it more difficult to achieve certain outcomes. To cite an extreme example, coercion may be unjustified, even though the patient chooses almost certain death when, with some forms of treatment, there is a prospect of survival. On the other side of the argument, there are outcomes, usually of a more highly "technical" nature, that are not readily defined as good in themselves. For example, there could be disagreement on how important it is to maintain a normal blood sugar level in diabetics. To take a broader view, the excessive emphasis on saving lives and reducing disability and pain has itself been criticized as inimical to even more important moral and spiritual values.[15] I cite these examples not to deny the greater ease with which outcomes can be accepted as desirable or undesirable in themselves, but to point out that even something as widely held to be true as this is, is subject to the rule that specific situations require specific decisions concerning the inherent validity of the measure. But a more significant limitation is that this kind of validity is only the first component – and not by any means the most important one – of a determination of the validity of the inferences concerning the quality of care.

Perhaps the most important single issue that comes under the heading of validity is the basis for asserting that certain processes lead to certain outcomes, or that any given outcome is the consequence of specified antecedent processes. Those who espouse the use of outcomes to assess the quality of care have argued, justifiably, that much of what is now accepted as good practice has no firm scientific foundation. This means that the causal linkage between process and outcome has not been securely established. They therefore conclude that since what might be called the "causal validity" of process measures is often doubtful, they have no choice but to use outcomes as measures of quality.[16] What they fail to realize is that causal validity resides neither in process nor in outcome, but in the link that joins them. In this respect there is perfect symmetry. To the extent that there are doubts about the causal linkage between given elements of process and given outcomes, the use of these elements as indicators of quality is of dubious value. But, for the same reason, the value of the use of these outcomes as indicators of quality is compromised to an equal degree. When the causal relationship between process and outcome is established, either can be used to make valid inferences about quality. When the causal relationship is not established, neither can be used. The state of medical science determines, with equal force, what elements of process or outcome can be used for what kinds of inferences about quality, and with what degree of certainty; and only scientific progress can improve the situation in this respect.

The presence of a valid causal linkage between specified processes and outcomes signifies only that it is possible to achieve certain outcomes under specified conditions. It does not mean that the outcomes observed in any given situation have been actually produced by the antecedent processes. For example, a patient may have improved spontaneously, without benefit of care; or he may have deteriorated in spite of treatment, because other factors have intervened. The consequences of care are very much influenced by the stage and the severity of illness, and by the physiological capacity of the patient to resist its ravages. The potential of the disease to cause harm, and that of the patient to resist it, are, in turn, influenced by many demographic, nutritional, psychological, environmental, and social factors. This means that when outcomes are used to make inferences about the quality of care, it is necessary first to establish that the outcomes can, in fact, be attributed to that care. We may call this the problem of "attribution," and its satisfactory solution may be said to confirm "attributional validity." Note that this kind of validity depends on the prior establishment of a causal linkage between process and outcome on scientific grounds. "Causal validity" refers to the capacity of specified processes to produce specified outcomes under specified conditions. Attributional validity refers to the inference that in any particular situation that capacity accounts for the actual observations.

Outcomes are particularly vulnerable to a loss of attributional validity mainly because intervening factors result in faulty specification of the conditions under which the process-outcome relationship has been measured. But, here also, one notes a curious symmetry between process and outcome. In the presence of causal validity one assumes that when appropriate care is given the desired outcomes will occur, with a pre-specified probability. Should one go beyond that by having to demonstrate that the expected outcomes have actually occurred and that they are actually attributable to prior care? Is there a "contributional validity" of process as an analogue to the "attributional validity" of outcomes? It seems to me that, in the abstract, the answer must be "Yes." But, in the course of assessment, the specification of the process usually includes the specification of the situation for which that process is appropriate. If this is well done, then there should be no problem with contributional validity. Unfortunately, the specification is not always sufficiently precise or complete. The specification of the patient's condition may be erroneous or insufficiently detailed, so that the relevance of the care provided is not fully established. As we shall see, this occurs frequently when criteria are developed for broad diagnostic categories. The specification of the process of care is incomplete when the entire process is not included in the assessment, so that departures from specification go unnoticed. For example, the adherence of the patient to the prescribed regimen is usually omitted from the assessment of quality. Less obvious is imperfect specification of the processes that are, ostensibly, included in the assessment. Say, for example, that surgery is appropriately recommended, and the appropriate operation is selected, but the procedure is poorly executed. The assessment of process will be faulty if it includes only surgical decision making and excludes surgical technique. Conversely, surgical technique may be immaculate, but the operation not indicated. By analogy, diagnostic tests may be indicated but improperly interpreted, or their findings not used, even though the tests are both indicated and reported correctly. I conclude that attributional validity cuts both ways, in that it applies to outcomes as well as to process, although the symmetry is not as precisely and logically determined as that for causal validity.

It is apparent that outcomes are not preferable to process when either causal or attributional validity is the basis for the comparison. There is perfect symmetry with respect to causal validity, and with respect to attributional validity I think the use of process usually has a slight edge. The advantage is increased, and the grounds for assessment radically altered, by the introduction of a new consideration which might be called "normative validity." The reasoning summarized by this term is that the practitioner is not responsible for the efficacy of the procedures he uses, but merely for selecting from what is available those procedures that are considered according to the best professional opinion to be the most efficacious. This means that process elements can still be used if there is general agreement that certain procedures are appropriate for certain situations, even though there is no "scientific proof" of appropriateness. "Normative validity" rests on the presence of professional consensus, so it could also be called "consensual validity." I use the former term because it can include other considerations in addition to consensus. For example, there may be no consensus, but there are, instead, two equally credible rival schools of thought. If the care given conforms faithfully to the recommendations of one or the other school, it could be considered to have an equal level of quality. The notion of normative validity also adapts easily to narrower definitions of the role of the practitioner or of the scope of assessment. For example, if the practitioner makes the correct diagnosis and prescribes the correct treatment, he may be said to have performed well, even though subsequent events over which he has much less control result in the treatment not being carried out as prescribed. The definition of the legitimate role of the practitioners and the legitimate scope of the assessment influence the normative validity of the inferences from the observation of certain aspects of process.

Validity is also influenced by the relevance of the chosen measures to the goals of care.[17] What I mean is perhaps best illustrated by a situation in which mortality rates are used to assess care when the purpose of care is only to reduce pain, discomfort, or anxiety. Obviously, the outcomes selected to assess the quality of care must be relevant to the objectives of that care.[18] But there is a question about whether the objectives in question are the ones that the practitioner has actually chosen or the ones that should have been chosen. It seems to me that both kinds of objectives should be used, because the use of each leads to valid inferences about different aspects of performance. Unfortunately, it is often difficult to reconstruct the intentions of the physician by a review of the record of care; and specifying what the objectives should have been requires knowledge not only of the technology of care, but also of the patient's situation and preferences, assuming an individualized definition of the quality of care has been adopted.

The incongruence between measures of quality and the objectives of care is easy to illustrate by means of outcome criteria. The problem seems less important in the assessment of process because the criteria of care, whether openly stated or only assumed, imply specification of relevance to some set of objectives. Unnecessary or redundant care, however, is obviously unrelated either to the actual or to the normative objectives of care. If a method of assessment simply takes account of the presence of needed care, without accounting for the presence of redundant care, to that extent it ignores the issue of relevance to objectives. When elements of process are to be assessed, there is the additional issue of the importance of these elements in the general scheme of care. Importance is perhaps a compound of the likelihood that a process element will have an effect, the magnitude of the effect, and the importance of the effect as a component of the patient's health and welfare. In some way, this complex of considerations is probably included in ratings of the importance of process criteria, a subject which will be described later in a subsequent volume of this work.

Outcomes are thought to be particularly vulnerable to misinterpretation due to inadvertent omission of the consequences of the entire range of alternative actions. A couple of examples will clarify this point. When two surgeons use the same operation, but one has a higher mortality rate than the other, it is necessary, as I have already pointed out in my discussion of attributional validity, to correct for differences in the characteristics of the patients and of their illnesses. But when, given comparable patients, one surgeon uses a procedure that has a higher mortality, whereas another uses one with lower mortality, a comparison of relative quality is not possible without information about the fate of patients who are not operated upon by each of the two surgeons. The second of these two examples involves an error of interpretation that comes from partial inclusion, and which can be corrected only if all alternative actions are accounted for, among them not doing anything. Of course, the general principle also applies to the consequences of nonsurgical treatment. Most probably it applies in the assessment of process as well. Consider a method of assessment based on an evaluation of the management of cases with a given diagnosis. Missing from this picture are all the cases of patients who should have had this diagnosis but were classified under another heading. At the program level, the cases included would be those who received care, whereas those excluded would be those who received no care of any kind during any given period, even though they could have benefited from care.

Sensitivity and specificity are central to the validity of all measurement. The specificity of many outcomes as a basis for inferences about the quality of care tends to be low. This is because many factors other than medical care influence health in a general sense, and, more specifically, the response to care. Obviously, specificity depends on the prior establishment of causal and attributional validity. But even when an outcome can be attributed, at least in part, to prior medical care, there is the further difficulty of determining which elements of process contributed to the failure to achieve expected outcomes. This is an important defect when it is necessary to fix responsibility in order to improve performance. In other situations, when all that is needed is to establish the value or impact of health care, this problem of specific attribution is not important, and may even be an advantage. To say that a measure is not specific is to condemn it. It is, therefore, important to find another terminology in order to describe the advantages of nonspecificity. In this case, outcomes may be said to be inclusive and integrative. As a result of this inclusivity, many measures of health status are good indexes of the general conditions of life in a society, including the quantity and the quality of the medical care it provides. It is easier to accept infant mortality, for example, as a measure of the quality of life in a society, than it is to see it as a measure of the quality of medical care. Similarly, when the object is to determine the quality of the health services received by an individual or a group, irrespective of what these services have been, and of who has provided them, outcomes are the logical, and easy, choice. Moreover, not all outcomes are necessarily low in specificity. It is possible to develop process-specific outcomes. The most specific of these are likely to be physiological measurements that have a strong causal linkage to specified treatments and are close to them in time.

The sensitivity of outcomes as measures of the quality of care depends on their responsiveness to differences or changes in care. There are two things to consider: the frequency with which a change in outcome is observed (for the better or worse) and the magnitude of that change. If the change in outcome is small, it may elude measurement; if it is very infrequent it may escape notice, unless samples are large. But, in either instance, the problem may not be inherent in outcomes as a whole, but in the given outcome used to make inferences about the quality of care. Let us take the death in the hospital of an elderly person as an example. When fully established, death can be measured with great certainty, and it is always reported, at least under the circumstances that concern us. In that respect it is an excellent measure! But when this phenomenon, that offers no measurement problem whatsoever under the circumstances I have described, is used to draw inferences about the quality of prior care, it is found to have serious shortcomings as to specificity and sensitivity. It is not specific because many factors other than the quality of care affect it, and because we may not be able to say what element in care was responsible for it or contributed to it. It is insensitive if deaths are relatively infrequent or if care must be radically wrong before it causes death, or fails to avert it. Nevertheless, it is reasonable to assume that there are other disturbances of physiological status that occur more readily and more frequently, in response to smaller deficiencies in care. Obviously, these would be outcomes that are more specific, more sensitive, or both. These outcomes would seem to be the preferred measures for assessing the quality of care, but their use may present other problems. Information about them may be more difficult to get. They may be more difficult to measure accurately. They may also have a less direct relationship to functional changes that are meaningful to the patient. This last point suggests that when the measure of outcome has no inherent validity, its relationship to other, inherently valid, outcomes is an element that influences its specificity and sensitivity.

The specificity and sensitivity of elements of process that have no inherent validity when they are used to assess the quality of care must also depend on the relationship of these elements to desired outcomes, since this is the way I defined quality in the first place. If this is the case, it leads to the conclusion that the sensitivity and specificity of the elements of process vary depending on what outcomes are chosen as the objectives of care and the legitimate criteria of its success. And the relationship between process elements and outcome depends on causal validity, attributional validity, and relevance to the objectives of care. For example, earlier I argued that deaths are likely to be unspecific and insensitive measures of the quality of care because fatality is not easily influenced by care, and because fatality involves the influence of many factors other than care. But if the averting of death is the legitimate objective of care, we will find that many elements of process are neither specific nor sensitive predictors of this outcome. If my reasoning is correct, we have encountered, once again, the seemingly inexorable symmetry that ties process to outcome. The only advantage that process measures seem to have, in this context, is that certain adverse outcomes occur rather infrequently, whereas the processes that lead to these outcomes are frequent, so that they are less likely to be absent from small samples. But this imbalance can be redressed if the more proximate outcomes are chosen as evidence of quality. Moreover, the more catastrophic outcomes are useful measures because, though infrequent, they unmistakably call attention to themselves.

There is perhaps one aspect of validity in which the symmetry between process and outcome does not hold. This is the peculiar vulnerability of outcome measures to erroneous interpretation as a result of "paradoxical effects."[19] Very briefly, the observation that poor health is unusually pervasive in a given population group may be evidence of good medical care rather than bad. This paradox arises mainly in two situations. In one of these, under what may be called the "survival effect," the prevalence of disability is increased when chronically ill people of any age are enabled to live longer with their disabilities, and healthy people to live to an older age, at which time disability becomes more frequent. The other mechanism that will bring about the paradoxical situation is the "discovery effect." In this situation, when medical care is better, more disease and disability are discovered, documented, and reported. Unless allowance is made for these paradoxical situations through proper study design, good care is in danger of being labeled bad, and bad care good.

Analogous paradoxes may also arise in the assessment of process, though they may not be equally important or equally obvious. For example, I suspect that the more a practitioner does for his patient, and the more information he includes in the record, the more he exposes himself to errors of commission, and to the discovery of these errors. In general, the availability of better records is an invitation to formulate and apply more rigorous criteria of care, while the absence of such records forces the adoption of less demanding criteria. Obviously, it would be inappropriate to make comparisons under these circumstances.

Contribution to Innovation in Medical Care

When the causal relationship between process and outcome is scientifically established, either of the two may then be used as a measure of quality with equal assurance, provided one guards against the other errors that I discussed in the preceding section. When causal validity is in doubt, the position of the purist would be that neither process nor outcome can be used without serious risk of error. While, strictly speaking, this is true, the practical demands of quality monitoring require that something be done. Under these circumstances, some have maintained that the processes that represent normative clinical behavior can be used as interim criteria and standards of quality. Their argument is that the practitioner's obligation is fully discharged if he uses the procedures that are recommended by the best professional opinion. More than this he cannot do.

The opposing view is that, under these circumstances, the use of outcomes is the only feasible and safe alternative. To use process criteria and standards is to run the risk of perpetuating possible error. The incorporation of insufficiently validated prevalent practices into the formal criteria and standards of a quality monitoring system is to give them unwarranted authority, and to contribute to their persistence. Once established, such practices are not only less likely to be questioned, but, as Brook has pointed out, ethical considerations may make it impossible ever to subject them to testing under experimental conditions (Brook 1973, p.126). By contrast, the errors that may result from the use of outcomes are easier to accept. When outcomes are favorable, antecedent care may receive undeserved credit. At worst, this means that useless procedures or those that are only mildly harmful will appear to have been useful. But when outcomes are unfavorable, antecedent care is likely to be subjected to scrutiny, so that truly harmful procedures are more likely to be identified.

The relationship of quality assessment to innovation in medical care seems to be at the heart of this argument. Everyone agrees that in clinical research, the validity of elements of process can be accepted only if a clear relationship to desirable outcomes is established under adequately controlled conditions. The question is whether quality assessment and quality monitoring for administrative purposes also have a learning and innovative function. In my opinion, the answer is a qualified "Yes."

The use of process criteria fosters the spread of innovation to the extent that those responsible for quality assessment seek and adopt the best available opinion. The use of outcome criteria, when it is coupled with the actual examination of antecedent process, has two possible consequences. It may lead to the reassessment of process in the light of the best current knowledge. To that extent it contributes to the diffusion of innovation. If process already conforms to the "best" criteria and standards, the observation of unfavorable outcomes has an additional, and unique, contribution. It may lead to questions about the validity of what is considered to be the best current practice. I believe, however, that it is inappropriate, and even dangerous, to expect that the quality monitoring mechanism itself will provide the setting or the means for establishing the legitimacy of these questions or for seeking better methods of management. The validation of causal relationships between process and outcome requires a degree of rigor in research design, of precision in measurement, and of skill in analysis and interpretation that is almost never possible in an operational monitoring system (Cochrane 1972). And conclusions that flow from observations under less well-controlled conditions are likely to contribute as much to error as to enlightenment.

There is another kind of innovation that has to do not with the validity of the causal linkage between process and outcome, but with other aspects of their use as tools for assessment and monitoring. For example, one may wish to study the efficiency with which certain adverse outcomes or nonadherence to certain process criteria will lead to a distinction between cases where patients are judged to have received good or bad care when more definitive measures of quality are used. Judgments of quality in which outcome measures have been used may have to be compared with judgments that were made with process measures in the same cases. The costs of implementing alternative methods of monitoring may need to be compared. For studies such as these, operating systems of assessment and monitoring are, of course, the obvious sites.

Cost

Relative cost is an important practical consideration which has figured rather prominently in the arguments for or against the use of process or outcome in quality assessment and monitoring. Unfortunately, the debate is largely speculative, since good data on cost are hard to find. Accordingly, about all I can do in this section is to explain the nature of the argument without giving its conclusions.

In a consideration of cost a distinction is to be made between the cost of the method itself and the cost implications of its use in quality assessment and monitoring. The cost of the method includes the cost of developing criteria and standards, and of obtaining, processing, analyzing, and interpreting the information. So many factors influence these costs that there is no reason to believe that either process or outcome is generally costlier than the other. The answer would seem to depend on the details of each situation.

The cost implications of the method arise from the behavior that results, or is thought to result, from the use of one method as compared to another. In this respect, many critics, including myself, have argued that a method of assessment that requires adherence to process criteria is an invitation to greater use of services and higher costs (Donabedian 1976). By contrast, a method in which outcome criteria are used is thought either not to invite greater use of service or to be a real inducement to more economical use. In fact, the situation is much more complicated than it first appears to be, and it does not permit such easy generalization.

Much of the criticism of the wastefulness of process criteria is addressed not to the use of process, in general, but to the use of a particular method, which offers what has been called a "laundry list" of all the procedures that may be justified in cases that fall into a rather broad diagnostic category. Similarly, the advantages claimed for methods based on outcomes depend on the assumption that there is a prior reorganization of care so as to generate strong professional and financial incentives not to engage in wasteful care. Thus, while Brook argues that process criteria are an invitation to waste, Blum argues that they are an instrument of cost control at the expense of quality; and both are correct, since each has a different model of monitoring in mind (Brook 1973, Blum 1974). Similarly, it is reasonable to expect that an emphasis on outcomes in preference to "laundry list" criteria will encourage savings in prepaid group practice. But the use of outcomes to judge quality of care in a fee-for-service system, without an examination of the means that were used to achieve these outcomes, could very well have the contrary effect.

All this has to do with the relationship between quality monitoring and inefficient or wasteful care. There is yet another issue that is even more fundamental, although it is often either imperfectly articulated or actually disguised. This has to do with the level of quality that a society wishes or can afford to make generally available. Among the many critics of the use of process in quality assessment, Havighurst and Blumstein deserve credit for at least having made this argument clearly and openly. Consider the relationship between medical care services used and health benefits, as it was portrayed in Chapter One. When expert practitioners are asked to set the standards of care in terms of the services needed, they tend to include every last service that is expected to make every iota of difference to expected outcome. These are not unnecessary services, but services which have some usefulness, though the increment of benefit is small relative to the cost of the additional service. The result is that care is extremely costly overall, and a portion of it has very low returns compared to cost. Furthermore, since the final segment of the curve that relates services to benefits is probably very flat, there is no clear point which can be used to set a limit on the accumulation of recommended services.[20] According to my terminology, the argument is that process criteria and standards embody an absolutist definition of quality, which is inappropriate from the viewpoint of either the individual or society, or both.

I believe that this analysis is basically sound. What is sometimes missed is that, at least in the abstract, it applies to outcome criteria as well as it does to process criteria. If the standards for outcome are set very high, somewhere near the highest point of the curve that relates services to health benefits, we have the same consequences. The corresponding services will represent a level of care that is very costly and, in part, inefficient. In this regard there is perfect symmetry; and this is not surprising, since the issue, fundamentally, is the choice of an appropriate definition of quality rather than its translation into process or outcome criteria. Process criteria appear to be the culprit only because practitioners are more adept at translating their absolutist definition of quality into its process equivalents than they are at doing the same with its outcomes.

Timeliness

An important consideration for the choice of a method of assessment is the timeliness of the information it provides when compared to the uses for which the information is needed. If the purpose is to influence or regulate the conduct of patient care, the information has to be reasonably current. Otherwise, the opportunity for using it most effectively may be missed, and, in time, the information may be seen as no longer relevant. In this regard measures of process have an obvious advantage, whereas outcomes, by their very nature, require time to develop and become apparent. And the longer the time that has elapsed between the receipt of care and the measurement of outcome, the more opportunity there has been for extraneous factors to enter the picture, obscuring the causal relationship between process and outcome. Thus, both relevance and validity are attenuated by the passage of time.

Process lends itself easily to prospective, concurrent, and retrospective assessment for preventive, interventive, and remedial purposes, respectively. Retrospective assessment, the most usual form, is ordinarily based on a review of past care as documented in the medical record. The object is to learn from past experience, so that care in the future may be improved. It is also possible, though more difficult, to obtain information during the process of care, so that one can intervene if an erroneous or a dangerous course of action is being pursued. Prospective assessment is based not on actual care but on plans for future care, which may be approved or rejected. This form of assessment has a specifically preventive function, though the other types of assessment, either by causing intervention during the course of care or by resulting in the correction of past errors, also have an important preventive effect.

Admittedly, the assessment of outcome is almost always retrospective, and it is often attempted so early that the outcomes are not yet fully known or so late that the results have lost some of their usefulness. Of course, such failings are not inevitable; they can be corrected by careful selection of outcome and of study design. In an insightful analysis, Brook and his associates at the Rand Corporation have pointed out the need to understand the natural history of specific outcomes in clearly defined situations, so that the outcomes can be measured during those time periods following care when they are most sensitive and specific as measures of differences in the quality of antecedent care (Brook et al. 1977, pp.35–36). Unfortunately, little is known about the natural history of disease under optimal, and different levels of less than optimal, care, so that the data are seldom available for determining the most discriminating combination of the specified outcomes and the "time windows" during which it is best to measure those outcomes.[21]

While outcomes are often thought of as phenomena that occur subsequent to care, it should be remembered that changes in physiological, biochemical, and clinical indicators of health status are taking place continuously during the process of care. In fact, the clinical management of the patient is always monitored and guided by staff who give detailed attention to such changes. It is, therefore, rather surprising to find that the concurrent observation of such indicators, which fit well under the heading of "outcomes," has not been more often used as a method for monitoring the quality of care, the latter being defined as an administrative or organizational, rather than a clinical, function. In fact, in a recent review of the subject it is reported that "no examples of the use of outcomes for the dual purposes of noting clinical progress and assessing quality could be found in the literature." (Brook et al. 1977, p.19) But this deficiency seems to me to be no more than a reflection of technical difficulties, missed opportunities, or both. Conceptually, immediate and intermediate elements in the chain of outcomes are as open to assessment as the elements in the contemporaneous unfolding of the sequence of care.

It is clear that the retrospective and concurrent assessment of outcomes corresponds rather well to retrospective and concurrent assessment of process. Can the same be said of prospective monitoring? At first blush, it is difficult to see how there can be prospective monitoring of outcomes, since outcomes have to occur before they can be measured. But, strictly speaking, this objection also applies to process. Earlier in this section, prospective monitoring of process was considered possible only because it was made to apply to *plans* for care. One could argue, therefore, that an assessment of projected care with respect to its likely outcomes is a form of prospective monitoring of outcome. In my opinion, other methods of outcome assessment that have been classified as "prospective" do not completely qualify.[22]

A reasonable conclusion that might be drawn from this analysis is that process and outcomes do not differ so very much with respect to timeliness. Nevertheless, there are many outcomes that occur too late to be useful in quality assessment for administrative purposes, though they may be important in controlled trials that are meant to test the efficacy of alternative methods of treatment or the effects of alternative ways of organizing care (Brook et al. 1977, pp.16–18). This is because in such trials the effects of other variables can be more readily controlled, so that the problem of attribution is eliminated or greatly reduced.

Adverse outcomes that are delayed raise another problem in quality assessment. This is the ethical problem of not intervening earlier to prevent such outcomes. It seems to me that if such outcomes can be predicted with reasonable certainty by a timely examination of process, it would represent malfeasance not to do so, unless there is some insuperable barrier. It is true that intervention, after the event, may forestall or reduce the future incidence of such outcomes. But, in the meantime, an unjustifiable amount of potentially preventable harm may have been done. Fortunately, when such outcomes are serious and frequent, a telltale "pattern" of events is likely to be detected early. Another safeguard that is included in many quality monitoring systems is the review of every single case of serious misadventure that can possibly be related to concurrent or antecedent care.[23] But when this is done one needs to consider, as we shall see in the following section, how efficient this method is for separating questionable care from acceptable care.

Feasibility, Acceptability, and Effectiveness

Brook and his associates do us a service by reminding us how much of the choice between process and outcome depends on pragmatic considerations (Brook et al. 1976, pp.14–17). We have already discussed some of these factors under the headings of validity and cost. Briefly, the choice depends to a large extent on what data are readily available, on the cost of obtaining, processing, and analyzing data, and on the validity of the data. I shall have more to say about these matters in a subsequent volume. It is clear, however, that the method becomes more expensive and less feasible if it requires information that is not collected and used in the ordinary course of events. Information that requires finding, interviewing, and examining former patients is not only very costly, but also difficult to gather.

Another requirement for assessment is the detailed specification of the criteria and standards of process and outcome. This is a subject that will be discussed in a subsequent volume. Now, it is enough to say that physicians find it much easier to specify criteria and standards for the activities that make up care than to say precisely what outcomes should be achieved at specified time intervals following optimal and various levels of suboptimal care.

Still another, essentially pragmatic, consideration is what might be called the "screening efficiency" of the items of process or outcome selected as a means for monitoring care. In monitoring systems, such items are almost always used not as definitive measures of quality, but as a means for separating cases in which patients need no further attention from those that require scrutiny as to the quality of care they have received. The failure to make the distinction between final assessment and provisional screening seems to have caused the greatest misunderstanding in systems of monitoring where the analysts pride themselves on using outcomes in preference to process. It should be recognized that, in such systems, outcomes are often used not as final judgments on the quality of care but as triggers that initiate the review that leads to a final judgment. That review is often, exclusively or predominantly, an assessment of process; it is sometimes followed by a search for structural factors that may have contributed to the deficiencies in care.

Screening efficiency depends on the balance of two errors: that of failing to find cases in which the quality of care is below acceptable standards, and that of including cases in which the quality of care is acceptable. These considerations are another manifestation of the more general issue of specificity and sensitivity, except that they are here applied to the screening function of elements of process or outcome. Obviously, the cost of the monitoring system depends very much on the proportion of cases that are subjected to detailed review, justifiably as well as unjustifiably. Its effectiveness depends on what proportion of substandard cases is detected and what proportion missed. Acceptability and credibility of the system is also at issue, since practitioners will quickly lose confidence in a system that seems often to produce error, either because far too many cases are questioned unjustifiably, or far too many that should have been questioned are allowed to slip through.

The choice of approach to assessment, beyond being a matter of technical feasibility, is also related to the readiness with which practitioners and others accept the method and find its results to be persuasive, insofar as they lead to a judgment on the quality of care. The acceptability and the persuasiveness of the method, in turn, have an influence on how much attention practitioners, administrators, and others will give to the findings, and how seriously they will commit themselves to bringing about a change (Brook et al. 1976, p.16). Unfortunately, as we shall see, little is known about the effectiveness of various methods of monitoring the quality of care, and next to nothing about the specific effects of the use of process versus outcome criteria as the basic emphasis in the method for assessment. There are those who believe, however, that when physicians fail to achieve realistic goals that they themselves have set for their patients, they become much more willing to search in the antecedent process of care for those elements that may have produced that failure.[24]

Ethics, Values, and Social Policy

It is interesting to note that neither the use of process nor that of outcome is free from ethical problems. With the use of process criteria there is an ethical problem that arises from including procedures that are still "experimental," or from withholding care that is generally viewed to be useful, even when there may be no convincing evidence to support this view. When outcomes are used for monitoring the quality of care, an ethical problem arises if adverse outcomes are used to show an established pattern or a stable probability of occurrence, when, if the process of care had been monitored, an earlier intervention could have prevented those adverse outcomes.

In Chapter One I discussed the social policy considerations that pertain to the choice of an appropriate definition and level of quality. These are fundamentally independent of whether process or outcome is used to define and assess quality of care. There is, however, as I mentioned earlier in this chapter, a greater likelihood that the absolutist definition of quality will be reflected in process criteria than in measures of outcomes. For this reason, and because process and outcome have different ethical and technical vulnerabilities, inequities could arise if process criteria are used to assess the quality of care received by certain population groups, while outcome criteria are used for others.

Let me amplify. In recent years there has been a tendency to extol the virtues of using outcomes for quality assessment, with emphasis especially on the usefulness of the method when one's aim is to control the costs of care. Accordingly, there is pressure that organizations which are subsidized partly or wholly by public funds rely more heavily on measures of outcome, in place of the more traditional methods of monitoring quality in which process criteria are used. If this happens, there is a danger that people who use these sources of care will have to accept care that is of lower quality, for one or more of the following reasons. Services that are generally considered to be useful could be withheld under the pretext that they are not sufficiently validated. The outcome criteria could be set rather low. In some cases, some outcomes may not even get measured. If they are measured, intervention might not occur until a pattern of adverse outcomes becomes clearly established. Such a pattern might be obscured by the time it takes for outcomes to emerge, by turnover in the membership of health plans, by geographic mobility, and by defects in the very system of data collection and analysis. When adverse outcomes are noted it may be difficult to assign responsibility because many factors other than medical care influence outcomes, because plan enrollees may have participated in any given plan for a relatively short period of time, because people receive care from many sources, and because within a single institution many practitioners share in the provision of care.

Admittedly, this is an alarmist's catalogue of almost all the weaknesses that the monitoring of outcome is heir to. I could have constructed an entirely different scenario in which the proper application of outcome criteria would have assured superior care to those under its beneficent aegis. For, let me repeat, many of the weaknesses I listed are not inevitably associated with the monitoring of outcome; nor is the monitoring of process free of deficiencies. Nonetheless, being of a suspicious turn of mind, I cannot help but think that when we are told that the care received by certain people should be judged by its outcomes, it is also implied that with these people we can take liberties that others would not allow! But this paranoia is not essential to my argument, which is, simply, that when different methods of quality assessment are applied to different population groups, the particular strengths and limitations of each method may result in an inequitable distribution of the attention that is given to quality, or of quality itself. If quality monitoring is a good (or, for that matter, an evil), its social distribution is subject to the rules of equity by which a society agrees to live.

There is another consideration which can be discussed under the heading of policy because it deals with the relative influence of professionals and clients on the definition of quality and on its surveillance. An emphasis on process tends to give primacy to the practitioners who are the high priests in charge of its technical mysteries and who also generate and control the information needed to assess it. The inclusion of an assessment of outcomes relaxes this monopoly and allows, even requires, the client to enter the sacred precinct. The client is fundamentally interested in outcomes; he can understand their significance when they are expressed in functional terms, and he is often the primary source of information concerning them. The use of outcomes gives greater influence to the client's perspective in defining quality and facilitates the participation of clients in the effort to monitor and enhance the quality of care. Outcomes, as Marshall so persuasively argues, can be the rallying point for an effective alliance between client and practitioner in the pursuit of quality (Marshall 1977, pp.42–50). But all this is only part of the truth, since process and outcome seem constantly to resist complete separation. Those parts of the process of care which pertain to the client-practitioner interaction are not only accessible to assessment by the client, but the clients are the more authoritative sources of criteria, standards, and information concerning this segment of care. As to outcomes, only the most expert practitioners can define and measure those outcomes that involve fine distinctions in physiological, biochemical, or functional states. Moreover, for all outcomes, expert knowledge is needed to specify what changes in health status are possible, how large these are, when they can be best measured, and how. Furthermore, the assessment of outcomes will give no information about the acceptability to the client of the manner in which the outcomes have been attained, unless specific aspects of client satisfaction are included among the outcomes that are measured.

Summary and Conclusions

When I began writing this section on the choice of process or outcome as the primary approach to the assessment of quality I expected to generate a catalogue of strengths and weaknesses for each of the two approaches; and I thought that this exercise would then lead us to the conclusion that neither is clearly preferable to the other in any general sense, while each may be more or less suitable for a particular purpose in a specific situation. I believe that, in the main, I have done this. But, what seems to me to be the more striking result of the analysis is the discovery of a basic symmetry that bonds process to outcome, so that the properties of the two are often almost mirror images of each other. No doubt this is the result of the fundamental causal linkage, demonstrable or assumed, that ties process to outcome. As a result, one encounters the same features of an intellectual landscape whether one begins with process and proceeds to outcome, or reverses the journey, going back from outcome to process. The features one sees are viewed from a different angle and in a different order, but they are the same features nonetheless.

Of course, there are differences as well. Many of these differences arise not from fundamental generic distinctions between process and outcome, but from less basic attributes of the particular elements of process or outcome that are selected, and from the way they are used in quality assessment. Nevertheless, such differences are important in the design of a method for assessment or monitoring that is to be used in a specified setting for a particular purpose. For this reason, the following quick summary will be a handy refresher.

Elements of process have a number of advantages as indicators of the quality of care. Practitioners have no great difficulty in specifying the criteria and standards of good care, at least for technical management. Even when these criteria and standards are not fully validated, they can serve as interim measures of acceptable practice. Information about technical aspects of care is documented in the medical record and is, usually, accessible, as well as timely, so that it can be used for preventive and interventive purposes, if this is desired. The use of this information also permits specific attribution of responsibility, so that credit or blame can be more easily ascertained, and specific corrective action taken.

The major drawback in the use of process for the assessment of the quality of care is the weakness of the scientific basis for much of accepted practice. The use of prevalent norms as a basis for judging quality may, therefore, encourage dogmatism and help perpetuate error. Because practitioners prefer to err on the side of doing more than is necessary, there is a tendency toward overly elaborate and costly care.[25] In contrast to this overemphasis on technical care, the management of the interpersonal process tends to be ignored, partly because the criteria represent primarily the practitioner's concerns and partly because the usual sources of data give little information about the practitioner-patient relationship.

The use of outcomes in the assessment of quality also has both its advantages and its disadvantages. An important advantage, when the scientific basis for accepted practice is in doubt, is that the emphasis on outcomes tends to discourage dogmatism and to help maintain a more open and flexible approach to management. Under certain forms of practice this may help in the development of less costly, but no less effective, strategies of care. Another advantage is that outcomes reflect all the contributions of all the practitioners to the care of the patient. Thus, outcomes can provide an inclusive, integrative measure of the quality of care. Among the many factors reflected by this measure is the patient's own contribution to that care which, in its turn, may have been influenced by the nature of the relationship between the patient and the practitioners. A more direct assessment of the patient-practitioner relationship can be obtained by including aspects of client satisfaction among the measures of outcome.

As if to provide a counterweight to the foregoing advantages, several disadvantages limit the use of outcomes as measures of the quality of care. Even expert practitioners are often unable to specify the outcomes of optimal care, as to their magnitude, timing, and duration. When indicators of health status are obtained, it is difficult to know how much of the observed effect can be attributed to medical care, and even more difficult to pinpoint specific responsibility within the segment that can be attributed to medical care. The choice of outcomes that have marginal relevance to the objectives of prior care is an ever-present pitfall. Even when the relevant outcomes are selected, and their attribution to prior care is not in doubt, information about many outcomes is often not available in time to make it useful for certain types of monitoring. Waiting for a pattern of adverse outcomes to become established can also be questioned on ethical grounds. And, finally, an examination of outcomes without an examination of the means by which those outcomes are attained can, under some circumstances, result in a lack of attention to the presence of redundant or overly costly care.

The preceding listing of the advantages and disadvantages supports the conclusion that the choice of an approach to assessment should reflect the requirements of each particular situation.[26] For example, the need to have timely information about the conduct of care, information that also pinpoints responsibility for error, favors an emphasis on detailed elements of process, "procedural end points," and immediate, process-specific "mini-outcomes."[27] And since, at the present, the "mini-outcome" approach has not been well developed, the more feasible alternative is to rely heavily on the details of process. By contrast, the need to have measures of general program effectiveness leads to the choice of the more inclusive measures of health status, supplemented by more general measures of process, such as data on the initiation of care and use of service. Measures of access, utilization, and health status are particularly appropriate when a program's providers accept total responsibility for the health of a defined population over longer periods of time.

But all this is only illustrative. In my opinion, the fundamental conclusion of this analysis should be a distrust of generalities. When a method for assessment or monitoring is designed, each element that is selected to indicate quality, whether it is an aspect of process or of outcome, should be characterized with reference to the properties I have discussed in this section under the headings of validity, innovation, cost, timeliness, feasibility, and values. And this characterization should, itself, be evaluated with reference to the objectives of the method of assessment or monitoring, and the details of the setting in which it is to be introduced and used. But, now that I have arrived at this decision not to generalize, let me make a case for one recommendation that may seem to contradict the rule. Seeing how little we know about the relationship between process and outcome, and how fundamental this relationship is to the inferences that are to be drawn from the findings of any assessment, it is important, whenever possible, to use both process and outcome elements simultaneously in any method of assessment or monitoring. In this situation, the measures of outcome have several functions. First, they may be indirect measures of aspects of process which are assessed through their outcomes because these latter are easier to measure. Second, the outcomes may be supplementary or confirmatory measures of aspects of process which are also directly assessed by information about elements of process. In this role, the outcomes provide a second tier in the monitoring method, one that helps us test whether the elements of process continue to be properly specified and measured. Similarly, the measures of process enable us to keep an eye, as it were, on the corresponding measures of outcome. In this way, the design of the system incorporates checks on its own validity. Such measurement is not, however, intended to be a form of research; it is merely the use of known relationships between process and outcome to ascertain whether the monitoring system is measuring what it is supposed to measure. A third important, though much less fundamental, function of outcomes in a monitoring system is their use as screens to separate cases into those that require detailed assessment from those that do not. In fact, I believe this to be the major feature of "outcome-oriented" methods of assessment as currently constituted; and this leads us to a final observation. In any system of monitoring, the measurement of outcome is only the first step in a succession of activities. In order to take corrective action, one must dig back into the processes that led to the unwanted outcomes. The identification of the errors in process will, itself, often lead to an examination of the structural features that were responsible for, or contributed to, less than optimal behavior. These necessary activities reaffirm the interconnectedness, the wholeness, of the structure-process-outcome chain. And it is on this foundation that any approach to assessment and monitoring must finally rest.

Notes to Chapter Three

[1] The work of Lee and Jones in *The Fundamentals of Good Medical Care* was part of the celebrated series of publications produced by the Committee on the Costs of Medical Care. Lee and Jones defined good medical care as a prelude to specifying needs for care, from which they derived corresponding requirements for personnel and facilities. For a more detailed description and assessment of this feature of their work see Donabedian 1973, pages 596–604. The recent extension of this work by Falk and Schonfeld and their associates is also briefly described, on pages 604–7 of the same source.

[2] For a more closely detailed development of the notion of primary objective, second-order objectives, and instrumentalities see Donabedian 1972. In this paper I also offer a proposal for including changes in the social distribution of health as a measure of the effectiveness of care.

[3] Some of these considerations, which are discussed in the first chapter of this monograph in the section on Contextual Influences, had appeared earlier, particularly under the heading of "Levels of Concern," in Donabedian 1969 (pp.5–7).

[4] In spite of my having taken great pains to understand De Geyndt's formulation I must admit that some parts of it have remained unclear to me. I think, however, that I have represented correctly its major outlines. Robert Brook (1973) has, apparently independently, discerned the same relationships that I have found and presented in Table 3-1. Receiving confirmation from such an insightful scholar increases my confidence that I have interpreted De Geyndt correctly, at least in this respect.

[5] As my former students, and now as good friends and highly respected colleagues, both Freeborn and Greenlick are generous in their acknowledgment of the influence of my earlier work. The primary purpose of my current exposition is not to claim credit, but to help the reader understand the conceptual structure underlying this and other classifications. A secondary, but important, aim is to let the reader know about this excellent classification, which he may be able to use in its present form, or to modify so that it fits his own purposes.

[6] Steinwachs and Yaffe (1978) provide an interesting example of the concern of a prepaid group practice over timeliness "as one dimension of the process of care that has received little attention." In their formulation, untimely care includes not

only care that is administered too late, but also care that is begun too soon or is entirely unnecessary.

[7] Enough time for practitioners and patients to be together appears to be a key factor in the attainment of satisfaction by both parties. The provision of an unhurried patient-practitioner encounter was, I believe, central to the success of two carefully planned demonstrations reported by Silver (1963) and by Goodrich et al. (1970), respectively. Mechanic, in his studies here and abroad, has also found that physicians become disgruntled if they feel there is not enough time to do a good job (Mechanic 1970, 1975).

[8] Hulka and her coworkers, as part of their important work on assessing the quality of the patient-physician relationship, have identified awareness of the patient's concerns as an indicator of success in communication between patient and physician, and have offered a method for measuring the extent of awareness (Hulka et al. 1971).

[9] Starfield and her associates have used as a measure of continuity of care the extent to which physicians recognize during a visit the health problems that were identified during previous visits. They have also reported the effect of redesigning the medical record on the recognition of previously identified problems. See Starfield et al. 1976 and Simborg et al. 1976.

[10] The number of physicians and facilities involved in the care of a patient or during an episode of illness, especially when there are no referrals, has been used as a measure of the continuity of care by many investigators. See, for example, Pugh and MacMahon 1967, Mindlin and Densen 1969, Shortell 1976, and Bice and Boxerman 1977.

[11] See Note 9, above.

[12] The ability to name the physician responsible for one's care in a clinic or group practice has been used as an indicator of the nature of the patient-physician relationship; see, for example, Walker et al. 1964.

[13] I draw this image from Samuel Butler's *Erewhon*. There, the children of the future are believed to be already alive as ghostly figures in another realm, eager to be born, though to do so entails perseverance and pain.

[14] The secular trend is well illustrated by the types of guidelines that accompanied the three waves of solicitations in the EMCRO program: those for fiscal years 1972, 1973, and 1974. The EMCRO (Experimental Medical Care Review Organization) program was set up to encourage the formation of prototype organizations that would develop and test methods for assessing the quality of care. The earliest set of guidelines urged the use of explicit process criteria to assess the care that was provided by organizations that represented local physicians. Two short years later, the guidelines emphasized the assessment of impact on defined population groups; the assessment was to be conducted by the organizations that had the responsibility for the care of such groups. Besides a change in the method of assessment, this development represents a shift in what I have

called the level and scope of concern, from concern for the individual physician who cares for the individual patient, to concern for organizations that have responsibility for large population groups. (See Arthur D. Little 1976, pp.51–53.) As I will point out in the text below, there is an affinity between outcome assessment and the assumption of responsibility for a population group.

An example of a program that has presented itself as outcome-oriented, while playing down its heavy reliance on process assessment, is the PEP (Performance Evaluation Procedure) program that was developed under the auspices of the Joint Commission on Accreditation of Hospitals (Jacobs et al. 1976, pp.23–31, 33–49). It is true that the method provides for the notation of status at discharge, as well as the occurrence of deaths and complications. But the information on physical status is often used only to indicate readiness for discharge, whereas the presence of deaths and complications is used to initiate a review of the antecedent process of care. Other elements in PEP are the justification of admissions and discharges, the justification of the diagnoses, and the justification of the performance of surgery and other hazardous procedures. All of these could be seen either as assessments of process or as a melding of process and outcome assessment.

[15] For example, Ivan Illich (1976) has argued that the presumption that death must be averted and pain or suffering relieved, in all situations and at all cost, makes people unnecessarily dependent on medical care and reduces the capacity for moral and spiritual development.

[16] I must apologize for my introduction of new terms to describe the several aspects of validity. I have used different terms in order to emphasize the distinctions that I see. I have had to invent new terms, or to use existing terms in new ways, simply because I do not know what terms and conventions already exist in the literature on measurement. I am ready to be corrected and instructed by those of my readers who know more than I do about this subject.

[17] I cannot find a good short term to describe this phenomenon. "Objectival validity" occurred to me, but I thought it was too awkward an expression.

[18] This seemingly obvious condition was first brought to my attention by Herbert Klarman, in his comments on one of my earliest papers on the quality of care (Donabedian 1966).

[19] The importance of recognizing and allowing for paradoxical effects in program evaluation was clearly identified by Sanders in 1964. For a somewhat more detailed discussion see Donabedian 1972, pp.154–55.

[20] Havighurst and Blumstein call this rather flat stretch of the curve "the quality/cost no man's land," since it lies between clearly "necessary" and clearly "unnecessary" care (Havighurst and Blumstein 1975, Figure and text on page 17).

[21] Brook et al. use the delightful expression "time windows" to summarize their thinking on this matter.

[22] Williamson at one time used the term "prospective epidemiology" to describe a method which involves the setting of explicit goals for specified outcomes, and the review of care when these goals are not attained (Williamson 1971). Brook et

al. place this method of outcome assessment in their category of retrospective methods. In their category of prospective methods they include what I have described as concurrent assessment. They also include, but with reservations, studies that involve a baseline assessment of health status, which is reassessed after care has been given. I believe there is some justification for calling this last method "prospective," since part of the measurement occurs prior to care, in anticipation of an assessment of the effects of care (Brook et al. 1977, pp.17–21).

[23] A good example of such a system is the Performance Evaluation Procedure (PEP) that was developed under the auspices of the Joint Commission on Accreditation of Hospitals (Jacobs et al. 1976). This principle has already had almost universal prior application in the work of hospital committees that examine prenatal, maternal, postoperative and other mortality, postoperative complications, transfusion reaction, nosocomial infection, and the like.

[24] I believe that this is an important assumption in the use of the method developed by Williamson (1971), which is briefly mentioned in Note 22, and which will be described in a subsequent volume of this work.

[25] For an interesting discussion of the preference between errors of commission and errors of omission see Scheff, 1963 and 1964.

[26] I am happy to see that Brook et al. reach the same conclusion in their landmark study of outcome criteria. See Brook et al. 1977, pp.14–15.

[27] I hesitate to give additional ammunition to the many friends who like to rib me about my weakness for new words. But I think that it would be convenient if we could indicate easily the differences between the more general measures of health status which take time to develop and which represent the sum total of many influences, and the more sensitive and specific changes in physiological and biochemical function that occur rapidly, almost in conjunction with the features of care that are responsible for them. Perhaps the former could be called "macro-outcomes," while the latter could be called "micro-outcomes" or "mini-outcomes." I hope that some of my readers will pursue this thought so that better words may be found.

References to Chapter Three

Arthur D. Little, Inc., *EMCRO—An Evaluation of Experimental Medical Care Review Organizations. Volume I: Executive Summary of Final Report.* Hyattsville, Maryland: National Center for Health Services Research, Division of Health Services Evaluation, 1976. 237 pp.

Bice, T.W., and Boxerman, S.B., "A Quantitative Measure of Continuity of Care." *Medical Care* 15 (1977):347–49.

Blum, H.L., "Evaluating Health Care." *Medical Care* 12 (1974):999–1011.

Brook, R.H., "Critical Issues in the Assessment of Quality of Care and Their Relationship to HMOs." *Journal of Medical Education* 48 (1973):114–34.

————; Davies-Avery, A.; Greenfield, S.; Harris, L.J.; Lelah, T.; Solomon, N.E.; and Ware, J.E., Jr.; *Quality of Medical Care Assessment Using Outcome Measures: An Overview of the Method.* Santa Monica, California: The Rand Corporation, 1976. 166 pp.

————; Davies-Avery, A.; Greenfield, S.; Harris, L.J.; Lelah, T.; Solomon, N.E.; and Ware, J.E., Jr.; "Assessing the Quality of Medical Care Using Outcome Measures: An Overview of the Method." *Supplement to Medical Care* 15 (1977):1–165.

Cochrane, A.L., *Effectiveness and Efficiency: Random Reflections on Health Services.* London: The Nuffield Provincial Hospital Trust, 1972. 92 pp.

De Geyndt, W., "Five Approaches for Assessing the Quality of Care." *Hospital Administration* 15 (1970):21–42.

Doll, R., "Surveillance and Monitoring." *International Journal of Epidemiology* 3 (1974):305–14.

Donabedian, A., "Evaluating the Quality of Medical Care." *Milbank Memorial Fund Quarterly* 44 (1966):166–203.

————, "Promoting Quality through Evaluating the Process of Patient Care." *Medical Care* 6 (1968):181–202.

————, *A Guide to Medical Care Administration, Volume II: Medical Care Appraisal—Quality and Utilization.* New York (now Washington, D.C.): American Public Health Association, 1969. 176 pp.

————, "Models for Organizing the Delivery of Personal Health Services and Criteria for Evaluating Them." *Milbank Memorial Fund Quarterly* 50 (1972): 103–54.

————, *Aspects of Medical Care Administration: Specifying Requirements for Health Care.* Cambridge, Massachusetts: Harvard University Press, for the Commonwealth Fund, 1973. 649 pp.

————, "Measuring and Evaluating Hospital and Medical Care." *Bulletin of the New York Academy of Medicine* 52 (1976):51–59.

Dror, Y., *Public Policymaking Reexamined.* San Francisco: Chandler Publishing Co., 1968. 370 pp.

Freeborn, D.K., and Greenlick, M.R., "Evaluation of the Performance of Ambulatory Care Systems: Research Requirements and Opportunities." *Supplement to Medical Care* 11 (1973):68–75.

Goodrich, C.H.; Olendzki, M.C.; and Reader, G.G.; *Welfare Medical Care: An Experiment.* Cambridge, Massachusetts: Harvard University Press, 1970. 343 pp.

Havighurst, C.C., and Blumstein, J.F., "Coping with Quality/Cost Trade-Offs in Medical Care: The Role of PSROs." *Northwestern University Law Review* 70 (1975):6–68.

Hulka, B.S.; Kupper, L.L.; Cassel, J.C.; and Thompson, S.J.; "A Method for Measuring Physicians' Awareness of Patients' Concerns." *HSMHA Health Reports* 86 (1971):741–51.

Illich, I., *Medical Nemesis: The Expropriation of Health.* New York: Pantheon Books, 1976. 294 pp.

Jacobs, C.M.; Christoffel, T.H.; and Dixon, N.; *Measuring the Quality of Patient*

Care: The Rationale for Outcome Audit. Cambridge, Massachusetts: Ballinger Publishing Co., 1976. 183 pp.

Lane, D.S., and Kelman, H.R., "Assessment of Maternal Health Care Quality: Conceptual and Methodologic Issues." *Medical Care* 13 (1975):791–807.

Lee, R.I., and Jones, L.W., *The Fundamentals of Good Medical Care.* Chicago: The University of Chicago Press, 1933. 302 pp.

Makover, H.B., "The Quality of Medical Care." *American Journal of Public Health* 41 (1951):824–32.

Marshall, C.L., "Quality in Medical Care: Consumerism and Caduceus." In *Toward an Educated Health Consumer: Mass Communication and Quality in Medical Care,* pp.33–53. Washington, D.C.: U.S. Government Printing Office, DHEW Publication No. (NIH) 77–881, 1977. 63 pp.

Mechanic, D., "Correlates of Frustration among British General Practitioners." *Journal of Health and Social Behavior* 11 (1970):87–104.

————, "The Organization of Medical Practice and Practice Orientations among Physicians in Prepaid and Nonprepaid Primary Care Settings." *Medical Care* 13 (1975):189–204.

Mindlin, R.L., and Densen, P.M., "Medical Care of Urban Infants: Continuity of Care." *American Journal of Public Health* 59 (1969):1294–1301.

Pugh, T.F., and MacMahon, B., "Measurement of Discontinuity of Psychiatric Inpatient Care." *Public Health Reports* 82 (1967):533–38.

Sanders, B.S., "Measuring Community Health Levels." *American Journal of Public Health* 54 (1964):1063–70.

Scheff, T.J., "Decision Rules, Types of Error and Their Consequences in Medical Diagnosis." *Behavioral Science* 8 (1963):97–105.

————, "Preferred Errors in Diagnosis." *Medical Care* 2 (1964):166–72.

Sheps, M.C., "Approaches to the Quality of Hospital Care." *Public Health Reports* 9 (1955):877–86.

Shortell, S.M., "Continuity of Medical Care: Conceptualization and Measurement." *Medical Care* 14 (1976):377–91.

Silver, G.A., *Family Medical Care: A Report on the Family Health Maintenance Demonstration.* Cambridge, Massachusetts: Harvard University Press, 1963. 359 pp.

Simborg, D.W.; Starfield, B.H.; Horn, S.D.; and Yourtee, S.A.; "Information Factors Affecting Problem Follow-up in Ambulatory Care." *Medical Care* 14 (1976):848–56.

Simon, H.A., *Administrative Behavior.* New York: The Macmillan Company, 1961. 259 pp.

Starfield, B.H.; Simborg, D.W.; Horn, S.D.; and Yourtee, S.A.; "Continuity and Coordination in Primary Care: Their Achievement and Utility." *Medical Care* 14 (1976):625–36.

Steinwachs, D.M., and Yaffe, R., "Assessing the Timeliness of Ambulatory Care." *American Journal of Public Health* 68 (1978):547–56.

Walker, J.E.C.; Murawski, B.J.; and Thorn, G.W.; "An Experimental Program in Ambulatory Medical Care." *New England Journal of Medicine* 271 (1964): 63–68.

Williamson, J.W., "Evaluating Quality of Patient Care: A Strategy Relating Outcome and Process." *Journal of the American Medical Association* 218 (1971): 564–69.

―――, *Assessing and Improving Health Care Outcomes: The Health Accounting Approach to Quality Assurance.* Cambridge, Massachusetts: Ballinger Publishing Company, 1978. 327 pp.

Appendix A

A More Detailed Specification of the Quality of Care Perceived as Normative Behaviors and Relationships, as Proposed by Donabedian (1968)*

I. Physician Behavior
  A. Technical Management of Health and Illness
    1. Adequacy of diagnosis
      a. Skill and discrimination in obtaining appropriate and complete information using the requisite clinical, laboratory, and other diagnostic techniques
      b. The use of valid information (accurate diagnostic tests) or inferences (e.g., from physical examination)
      c. Sound judgment in evaluating the information obtained
      d. Completeness in evaluating the information obtained
      e. Validity of diagnosis
    2. Adequacy of therapy
      a. Choice of effective and specific therapeutic regimen prescribed with due regard to expected risks arising from therapy and the condition to be treated
      b. Adequate management of pain, discomfort, and distress without undue prejudice to the diagnostic process
      c. Informing the patient about risks and side effects associated with treatment
      d. Maintaining adequate surveillance with the object of reducing risks and maximizing benefits
    3. Parsimony or minimum redundancy in diagnostic and therapeutic procedures (The issue of efficiency in terms of the economic use of

---

* Donabedian, A., "Promoting Quality through Evaluating the Process of Patient Care." *Medical Care* 6 (1968):181–202.

resources, although an important factor in the organization of medical care, will not be considered here. The emphasis will be on the logical necessity to have certain items of information and the therapeutic necessity to use certain treatments.)

4. Full exploitation of medical technology
   a. Maximum effectiveness in applying existing technology; knowledge of the technology and skill in its application
   b. Discrimination in the introduction and utilization of new technology
   c. Discrimination in discarding old methods

5. Full exploitation of professional and functional differentiation; recognition by the physician of his own limitations and the use of other specialists and of other professions where the need arises

B. Socioenvironmental Management of Health and Illness
   1. Attention to social and environmental factors, especially within the family and at work, having relevance to the following:
      a. Identifying and eliminating barriers to seeking and maintaining care
      b. Arriving at the professional definition of need
      c. Adjusting the frequency and content of the periodic review of all "well" persons
      d. Obtaining and evaluating information in the diagnostic process
      e. Planning and recommending treatment

   2. Use of larger social units (usually the family) as the units of care wherever appropriate in terms of:
      a. Therapeutic manipulation of social and environmental factors in the interests of the individual patient
      b. Using the larger unit as an object of care — for example, in considering the family epidemiology of infectious disease and the social impact of long-term illness on the family

   3. Use of community resources on behalf of the patient

   4. Attention to broader community interests — for example, in the reporting of communicable diseases

C. Psychological Management of Health and Illness
   1. Attention to psychological and emotional factors in:
      a. Identifying and eliminating barriers to seeking and maintaining care
      b. Arriving at the professional definitions of need
      c. Adjusting the frequency and content of the periodic review of "well" persons
      d. Obtaining and evaluating information in the diagnostic process
      e. Planning and recommending treatment

D. Integrated Management of Health and Illness
   1. Periodic review of "well" persons with special attention to promotion of mental and physical health; the early detection of physical and emotional deviations, through the use of appropriate screening mechanisms; and the use of appropriate primary preventive techniques for illness, accidents, injury, behavioral and emotional problems, etc.
   2. Using visits for the care of illness as occasions for the management of health
   3. Adequate follow-through on suspected abnormalities or health problems
   4. Identification of "high-risk" situations and appropriate adaptation of the amount and content of health management and medical care of such risk
   5. A developmental and anticipatory or interceptive orientation in the management of health and illness with due attention to preventing physical, social, and behavioral breakdown
   6. Attention to rehabilitation and restoration of function

E. Continuity and Coordination in the Management of Health and Illness
   1. Continuity and coordination of care for individual patients through either the establishment of a personal relationship with one physician or the coordination of care provided by several physicians, or both mechanisms
   2. Adequacy of the individual patient record and its ready availability as the major tool of coordination and continuity of care
   3. Continuity and coordination of care for several or all members of a family and the availability of family health records to the treating physician

II. The Client-Provider Relationship
   A. Some Formal Attributes of the Client-Provider Relationship
      1. Congruence
         Similarity of physician and patient expectations, orientations, etc.
      2. Adaptation and flexibility
         The ability of the physician to adapt his approach not only to the expectations of the patient (for greater or less affectivity, for example) but also to the demands of the clinical situation in terms of greater or less control, greater or less reciprocation of emotional involvement, and so on
      3. Mutuality
         Gains for both physician and patient
      4. Stability
         A stable relationship between patient and physician

B. Some Attributes of the Content of the Provider-Client Relationship

   1. Maintenance of maximum possible client autonomy, and freedom of action and movement (especially critical for institutionalized patients)

   2. Maintenance of family and community communication and ties (especially critical for institutionalized patients)

   3. Maximum possible degree of egalitarianism in the client-provider relationship

   4. Maximum possible degree of active client participation through
     a. Sharing knowledge concerning the health situation
     b. Shared decision making
     c. Participation in carrying out therapy

   5. Maintenance of empathy and rapport without undue emotional involvement of the provider

   6. Maintenance of a supportive relationship without encouragement of undue dependency

   7. Maintenance of a neutral, noncondemnatory attitude towards moral and other values of the client

   8. Confining provider influence and action within the boundaries of his legitimate social functions

   9. Avoidance of exploitation of the client economically, socially, sexually, etc.

  10. Maintenance of client dignity and individuality

  11. Maintenance of privacy

  12. Maintenance of confidentiality

Appendix B

Classification and Listing of Information To Be Used in Assessment of the Quality of Care, as Proposed by Donabedian (1968)*

I. Characteristics of the Settings within Which the Medical Care Process Takes Place (Structure)

It is assumed that good care is more likely to be provided when the settings are favorable, and that we know what constitutes a "favorable" setting.

A. Physical Structure, Facilities, and Equipment

1. Presence or absence of certain facilities and equipment in relation to specific care functions

2. Space and physical layout in relation to function

B. General Organizational Features

1. Ownership and auspices

2. Profit or nonprofit status

3. Accreditation, affiliation, and residency approval status

4. Other interinstitutional functional relationships (for example, as part of a regionalization program)

5. Group practice, partnerships, "solo" practice

C. Administrative Organization

1. Boards of trustees: their composition and activities

2. Administrator: qualifications and relationships with board and staff

---

* Donabedian, A., "Promoting Quality through Evaluating the Process of Patient Care." *Medical Care* 6 (1968):181–202.

To maintain the historical perspective, I am presenting the classification in its original form, even though I would now prefer to place many of the items that are listed under "client behaviors" in the category of "outcomes." I would also exclude "satisfaction of health professionals" from the category of outcomes, for reasons described in Chapter One. The reasons for the ambiguity in classifying "use of service," as well as for that in some other items in this list, are discussed in Chapter Three.

D. Staff Organization
   1. Qualifications: formal degrees, certification, experience, etc.
   2. Number of staff related to work load
   3. Staff organization and policies governing staff activities
      a. Educational functions: maintenance and promotion of staff competence
      b. Control functions: utilization review, various types of audits of staff performance, etc.

E. Fiscal and Related Aspects of Organization
   1. Hospital accommodation
   2. Source of payment of bill and extent of patient participation in payment

F. Geographic Factors; distance, isolation, etc.

II. Characteristics of Provider Behavior in the Management of Health and Illness (Process)
It is assumed that there are acceptable standards of what constitutes "goodness," and that good care makes a difference in terms of health outcomes.
   A. Extent to Which Screening and Case-Finding Activities Are Carried Out
      1. Routine procedures applicable to the older age group: examples are activities for the detection of glaucoma, diabetes, cervical cancer in women, lower bowel cancer, breast cancer, visual and hearing defects
      2. Screening and case-finding activities related to special-risk situations: examples are bleeding from the rectum (sigmoidoscopy); blood in the urine (cystoscopy); indigestion (barium meal and occult blood); hypertension (eyegrounds, urine, catecholamines, etc.)
      3. Follow-up on "red flag" findings with appropriate diagnostic and therapeutic activities: examples are bleeding from body orifices; certain abnormal laboratory findings (urine or blood sugar, for example)

   B. Diagnostic Activities
      1. Diagnostic work-up
         a. Frequency of performance of specified test per unit population
         b. Diagnostic work-up for specified disease situations; volume and nature of tests, etc.
      2. Patterns of diagnostic categorization; completeness, exhaustiveness, specificity, etc.
      3. Validation of diagnosis
         a. Pathological examination reports on tissues and postmortem
         b. Preoperative versus postoperative diagnosis
         c. Admission and discharge diagnoses
      4. Validation of primary diagnostic information; special studies on accuracy of lab reports, interpretations of x-ray films, etc.

C. Treatment

1. Preventive management and supervision of certain diseases; minimal or optimal standards of number of visits or routine follow-up in given diseases such as diabetes, hypertension, syphilis, etc.

2. Patterns of use of drugs, blood, and biologicals in general
   Examples:
   a. Total prescribed drug utilization per capita and per 1,000 physician visits
   b. Use of antibiotics, especially in mixtures
   c. Use of antibiotics without testing for sensitivity of microorganism
   d. Use of "shot-gun" hematinics
   e. Use of multivitamins
   f. Use of tranquilizers
   g. Use of blood by amount of blood, age, sex, etc.; incidence of single-unit transfusions

3. Patterns of use of drugs, blood, and biologicals in specified diagnostic situations

4. Patterns of surgery
   a. Surgical rates by type of procedure, with emphasis on certain operations more open to abuse: examples are tonsillectomy, appendectomy, hemorrhoidectomy, varicose vein operation, and certain gynecological operations, including hysterectomy, supracervical hysterectomy, uterine suspension
   b. Patterns of multiple operations, including second operations suggestive of possible deficiencies in first operations
   c. Removal of normal tissue at operation

D. Consultation and Referral

1. Patterns of consultation and referral by category of physician making request, type of consultant, disease characteristics, patient characteristics, institutional settings, etc.

2. Consultations and referrals in specific disease situations, including emotional and psychiatric problems and referral to psychiatrists

E. Coordination and Continuity of Care
   Number of physicians, hospitals, and other providers involved in the care of a single patient over a period of time or during a single episode of illness or care

F. Use of Community Agencies and Resources
   Volume and patterns of use, in general and for specified conditions or situations

III. Other Provider Behaviors Possibly Indicative of Strength or Weakness in the Organization of Care
   A. Staff Turnover and Absenteeism

   B. Reporting Ill (for example, among nursing students)

C. Use of Health Services by Providers Who Are Presumably Informed about Sources of Good Care

IV. Client Behaviors Possibly Indicative of Defects in the Organization of Care or the Client-Provider Relationship (Process and Outcome)
A. Complaints: volume and type

B. Compliance and Noncompliance: broken appointments; noncompliance with therapeutic regimen (drugs, diet, rest or exercise, etc.); premature termination of care; discharge against advice

C. Knowledge
1. About health and illness in general
2. About current illness

D. Changes in Knowledge or Behavior Expected after Prior Exposure to Medical Care
For example: knowledge about prenatal and well-baby care resulting from having had a child; appropriate institution of prenatal and well-baby care

V. Characteristics of Use of Service (Process or Outcome)
Studies of the utilization of service have important implications for quality. Insufficient care means poor care. Similarly, unnecessary care is not only costly but can also denote poor quality — in surgery, for example. It is assumed that adjustments have been made for factors that influence utilization, other than patient care.
A. Volume of Care
1. Levels of utilization in the general population and population subgroups classified by age, sex, race, income, occupation, education, place of residence, insurance status, etc.

2. Components of the utilization rates: "initiation," proportion receiving one or more services; "continuation," number of services for those who receive one or more services

3. Use by place of care: office, home, hospital, nursing home, etc.

4. Use by source of care:
a. Type of health professional
b. Specialty status

VI. Characteristics of Health and Other Outcomes
It is assumed that adjustments have been made for factors that influence outcome, other than patient care.
A. Health Outcomes
1. General mortality, morbidity, and disability rates (The problems of interpretation would be very severe but one would examine secular trends, geographic variations, etc.)

2. Mortality in special subgroups
   a. Infant mortality and its components
   b. Maternal mortality
   c. Other age- and sex-specific mortalities

3. Mortality by cause

4. Longevity
   Life expectancy, general and at given ages

5. Composite indexes of illness or health giving average number of days lost from morbidity and mortality combined or the average number of remaining days after losses have been subtracted

6. The occurrence of preventable morbidity or disability in the general population (This approach is based on the assumption that, given good care, either currently or during years or decades preceding old age, some of the current morbidity and disability would have been prevented: examples are prevalence of iron-deficiency anemia; loss of vision due to glaucoma; loss of hearing due to middle-ear disease; rheumatic heart disease; diabetic acidosis; amputations in diabetics and other patients; stage and extent of cancer at time of diagnosis.)

7. The occurrence of certain complications of, or failures in, therapy: examples are decubitus ulcers; cardiac decompensation; incomplete control of diabetics

8. Case fatality rates and operative mortality rates, by type of illness or operation and type of provider, with corrections for demographic and socioeconomic characteristics of patients

9. The occurrence of specified complications during the course of care or following surgery — for example, postoperative infection

10. The restoration of physical function following certain traumatic or neurological diseases: examples are recovery after fractures; residual disability following strokes

11. Social restoration following mental illness: examples are ability to remain in the community (as indicated by readmission rates); ability to find and maintain employment

B. Satisfaction
   1. Patient satisfaction is not necessarily, nor even usually, an indicator of the technical quality of care, but attention to patient needs is an important aspect of care, and patient satisfaction an important objective, in addition to technical performance

   2. Satisfaction of the health professionals providing care (While this is a dimension that is seldom mentioned, it is reasonable to assume that the best technical care cannot be maintained if the persons who provide it are unhappy with the work they do and the conditions under which it is done.)

Appendix C

Classification and Listing
of Information To Be Used
in Evaluating the Performance
of Ambulatory Care Systems, as
Proposed by Freeborn and Greenlick (1973)*

I. Assessment of Effectiveness
   A. Technical Effectiveness
      1. Structure
         a. Physical structure, facilities, and equipment
         b. Range and scope of services
         c. General organizational features, such as ownership, accreditation, affiliation, and the role of the medical staff in the organization
         d. Administrative organization and policy-making structure
         e. Staff organization, such as numbers, types, and qualifications, as well as policies governing the staff
         f. Fiscal and related aspects of organization, such as financing, source, and method of payment
         g. Geographic factors, such as distance, isolation, and geographic availability and accessibility of services and facilities

      2. Process of Providing Care
         a. Accessibility
            (1) Definition of the population to be served or eligible for care, and its social and demographic characteristics (These data are essential to identify the population at risk and to provide a denominator for utilization and other rates.)
            (2) Social and demographic characteristics, by selected morbidity, mortality, and disability rates, and by utilization patterns

---

* Adapted from Freeborn, D.K., and Greenlick, M.R., "Evaluation of the Performance of Ambulatory Care Systems: Research Requirements and Opportunities." *Supplement to Medical Care* 11 (1973):68–75. Used with permission.

(These data aid in evaluating the relationship between need, as defined by disease patterns, and use of services.)

    (3) Population groups with identifiable diseases not yet diagnosed, or diagnosed but not yet under treatment (Such data assist in identifying unmet need.)

    (4) Utilization patterns by time, place, type of service, type of provider; by presenting and associated morbidity symptoms; and by episodes and procedures

  b. Provider performance

    (1) Data relating to the *volume of care*, including utilization of services in relation to need (expressed in terms of selected symptoms or morbidities)

    (2) The *extent of screening and case-finding*, as indicated by the number of routine procedures and services applicable to age and sex groups; extent of preventive services used in connection with treatment; screening and case-finding of high-risk groups; and appropriate follow-up on "red flag" findings

    (3) Data concerning the *adequacy of diagnostic work-up and treatment*, including patterns of completeness, and specificity of diagnoses; validation of primary diagnostic information (e.g., special studies on accuracy of laboratory reports); prevention, treatment, and rehabilitation of certain diseases; patterns of use of drugs, blood, and biologicals; consultation and referral patterns; and extent of duplication of laboratory, x-ray, and other tests and medications

  c. Continuity

    (1) Number of patients who have and use a central, coordinated source of care and/or a primary physician

    (2) Frequency and appropriateness of referrals and consultations; coordination in the use of resources outside the system

    (3) Degree of compliance, particularly with respect to high-risk patients (e.g., hypertensive patients)

    (4) Degree of follow-up on abnormal findings

 3. Technical Outcome of Care

  a. General mortality, morbidity, and disability rates over time

  b. Mortality in special subgroups (infant, maternal)

  c. Functional disability

  d. Occurrence of preventable morbidity or disability

  e. Restoration of physical function

  f. Restoration of social function

  g. Occurrence of specified complications of care

  h. Case-fatality rates for diseases and operations

  i. Occurrence of complications or failures in therapy

B. Psychosocial Aspects of Effectiveness

 1. Patient Satisfaction

a. Satisfaction with *accessibility* as indicated by attitudes and knowledge regarding:
   (1) The extent to which services are available at the time and place needed
   (2) The ease of obtaining services, both for regular appointments and emergencies
   (3) The degree to which the patient understands how the system operates and the benefits and services available
b. Satisfaction with *quality of care* as indicated by attitudes toward:
   (1) The level of technical proficiency or competence of the patient's physician or other health personnel contacted by the patient
   (2) The outcome of illness — whether the patient perceives a change in his condition as a result of care
c. Satisfaction with *process of care and interpersonal relationships* as determined by measuring:
   (1) The extent to which patients value the availability of a primary care physician or central source of care
   (2) The perception of the physician's and other personnel's interest and concern
   (3) The degree of trust and confidence in the physician
   (4) The degree of understanding of the condition or diagnosis
   (5) The extent to which there is difficulty understanding the physician's instructions or other aspects of the treatment plan
d. Satisfaction with *system arrangements*
   (1) As ascertained by attitudes toward:
       (a) Physical surroundings and facilities
       (b) Patient flow, including appointment system; waiting time and use of time once in the system; helpfulness of personnel; and mechanisms used for solving problems and complaints
       (c) Scope and nature of benefits and services offered
   (2) As indicated by behavior observations that include:
       (a) Extent of medical care use outside the system
       (b) Proportion of subscribers who leave the program and choose other health plans
       (c) Number and type of complaints received by the medical care system
       (d) Broken appointment and cancellation rates
       (e) Rates of compliance with prescribed regimens
       (f) Proportion of patients who change physicians, assuming there is choice available within the system
2. Provider Satisfaction
   a. As indicated by staff attitudes and perceptions with respect to the following factors:
       (1) Autonomy/Organizational Control

       (a) Satisfaction with pace of work and control of pace of work
       (b) The extent to which staff can define and determine what is technically needed without organizational influence, and the degree to which staff can fully use their special skills and knowledge
       (c) Satisfaction regarding adequacy of resources for provision of care
       (d) Satisfaction with the degree of control over the scope and content of staff work
       (e) Satisfaction with type of supervision
    (2) Patient/Staff Interaction and Staff Relationship
       (a) The ease or difficulty of staff relationships with patients, and the extent to which the organization affects such relationships
       (b) The extent to which professionals feel they have the necessary time to spend with patients and thus to practice good quality medical care
       (c) Satisfaction regarding relationships with other staff members, including the administration
    (3) Prestige/Status
       (a) Satisfaction with opportunities to improve knowledge and skills and to advance within the organization or profession
       (b) Satisfaction with pay, fringe benefits, and working conditions
       (c) General opinions and evaluation of the desirability of the setting as a place of work, compared to other settings in the health field
       (d) Evaluation of the organization's ability to survive in its environment, its future chances for growth and success, and its prestige and status in the broader health community
  b. Other indications of staff satisfaction or dissatisfaction with the system, including turnover rates, absenteeism, excessive use of sick leave, and quality of work

II. Assessment of Efficiency
   ...In evaluating the relative efficiency of alternative systems of health care delivery, both the production function (the relation between output and input) and the cost function (the relation between costs and output) must be examined. Estimation of the production and cost functions may permit identification of a more efficient mix of the services and resources required to meet the needs of the population at risk. In general, the minimum data required to develop these functions include:

  A. Cost data: salary schedules; capital and equipment costs; maintenance costs; costs of supplies; costs per patient per year; costs per family per year; and costs per unit of service

B. Productivity data: numbers of patients seen and services rendered; number and type of personnel; daily work loads; activities performed by personnel and time involved; and procedures for scheduling patients

C. Population characteristics and morbidity data (so that above measures of cost and productivity can be standardized by age, sex, and case-mix)

Appendix D

Classification and Listing
of Information (Obtained from
Specified Sources) To Be Used in
Assessment of the Quality of Maternal
Care, as Proposed by Lane and Kelman (1975)*

I. Prevention
   A. Prenatal
      1. Obtaining family history (P,R)
      2. Obtaining menstrual history (P,R)
      3. Obtaining past medical (including surgical) history (P,R)
      4. Obtaining past pregnancy history (P,R)
      5. Obtaining present pregnancy history (P,R)
      6. General physical examination (P,R)
      7. Pelvic examination and evaluation of the status of the current pregnancy (P,R)
      8. Clinical pelvimetry (P,R)
      9. CBC (or Hb or HCT, WBC, and differential) (P,R)
     10. Urinalysis (P,R)
     11. Standard test for syphilis (P,R)
     12. Blood grouping and Rh typing (P,R)
     13. Rubella antibody screening (P,R)
     14. Pap smear (P,R)

---

* Adapted from Lane, D.S., and Kelman, H.R., "Assessment of Maternal Health Care Quality: Conceptual and Methodologic Issues." *Medical Care* 13 (1975):791–807. Used with permission.

Letters in parentheses indicate the source of the information as follows: (C) consumer interview, (H) hospital site schedule, (P) prenatal/postpartum site schedule, and (R) medical record abstract.

15. Pregnancy test if indicated (P,R)
16. Immunizations (P,R)
17. Prenatal classes (P,R)
18. Interval visit histories (P,R)
19. Monitoring weight (P,R)
20. Monitoring blood pressure (P,R)
21. Monitoring urinalysis (P,R)
22. Recording uterine size (P,R)
23. Recording time fetal movements first felt (P,R)
24. Auscultation for FHT after quickening (P,R)
25. Recording presentation (P,R)
26. Pelvic examination after 36 weeks to determine the effacement and dilation of the cervix (P,R)
27. History of preconception care (P,C,R)
28. Planned or unplanned pregnancy (P,C,R)
29. Contraceptive practices (R)
30. Month of gestation prenatal care initiated (C,R)
31. Assessment of patient's level of understanding and knowledge of maternity process, and related educational factors (P,R)
32. Counseling on gestation and labor (P,C)
33. Use of appropriate literature (P,C)
34. Information or discussion of program facilities, and utilization, e.g., keeping appointments, when to call, hospital tour (P,C)
35. Number of prenatal appointments (P,R)

B. Labor and Delivery
    1. Obtaining menstrual history (R)
    2. Obtaining previous obstetric history (R)
    3. Obtaining history of abdominal pain and uterine contractions (R)
    4. Obtain admission blood pressure (R)
    5. Determine fetal position (R)
    6. Follow uterine contractions, abdominal, or uterine pain (R)
    7. Auscultate fetal heart tones (R)
    8. Determine extent of bleeding (R)
    9. Determine condition of cervix and membranes (R)
    10. Clinical pelvimetry (unless performed previously) (R)
    11. CBC (or Hb or Hct, WBC, and differential) (H,R)
    12. Urinalysis (H,R)
    13. Blood type and Rh if not already determined (R)

14. Type of delivery (R)
15. Episiotomy (R)
16. Observation first hour after delivery (H)
17. Instructions in perinatal care (H,C,R)
18. Instruction in infant care and feeding (H,C)
19. Instruction in family planning (H,C)
20. Apgar scoring (H,R)
21. Initial examination newborn (H,R)
22. PKU (R)
23. Infant eye prophylaxis (R)
24. Vit K oxide to infant (R)
25. Referral for well-baby care (H)
26. RhoGAM (R)
C. Postpartum
　1. Obtaining menstrual history (R)
　2. Obtaining past pregnancy history (R)
　3. Obtaining previous contraceptive history (P,R)
　4. Obtaining social and sex history (R)
　5. Interval history and symptoms (P,R)
　6. Pap smear (P,R)
　7. General physical examination (P,R)
　8. Pelvic and breast examination (P,R)
　9. Instruction in breast self-examination (P,R)
　10. Discussion of choices of family planning methods (P,R)
　11. Instruction in use of selected family planning method (P,R)
　12. Return for postpartum visit (R)
　13. Return for interconceptional care (R)
II. Minimization of Adverse Consequences
A. Prenatal
　1. Identification menstrual abnormality (R)
　2. Identification abnormal reproductive history (R)
　3. Identification abnormal family or father's history (R)
　4. Identification pre-existing disease having relevance to present pregnancy (e.g., diabetes, hypertension, tuberculosis, syphilis) (R)
　5. Identification previous surgical procedures (R)
　6. Identification malnourished patient (R)
　7. Identification of excessive or insufficient weight gain (R)
　8. Identification of individual exposed to Rubella (R)

9. Identification of abnormal presentation (R)
10. Identification of abnormal Pap smear (R)
11. Identification of abnormal physical findings (R)
12. Monitoring of glycosuria or proteinuria (R)
13. Monitoring of elevated blood pressure (R)
14. Monitoring of edema (R)
15. Performance of atypical antibody screen in Rh negative patient (R)
16. Identification of antibody and zygosity of father when maternal atypical antibody present (R)
17. Performance of antibody titer every four weeks when maternal antibody present (R)
18. Performance of amniocentesis when titer is 1:8 or more (R)
19. Identification of anemic patient (R)
20. Identification of patient with urinary tract infection (R)
21. Identification of other complications of present pregnancy (R)
22. Performance of supplemental tests or procedures consistent with the diagnosis (e.g., culture and sensitivity, glucose tolerance test, chest x-ray, sickle prep, etc.) (R)
23. Management of diagnosed conditions: medications, monitoring, counseling (R)
24. Referrals (P,C,R)
25. Recommended modification of behavior (e.g., smoking withdrawal) (P,C,R)
26. Change in status of maternal health problem (C,R)
27. Hospitalizations during present pregnancy (C,R)

B. Labor and Delivery
   1. Obtaining previous surgical history (R)
   2. Identification complicated pregnancy (R)
   3. Identification prolonged rupture membranes (R)
   4. Identification abnormal presentation (R)
   5. Identification uterine dysfunction (R)
   6. Identification other complications of labor and delivery (R)
   7. Induction (R)
   8. Stimulation of labor (R)
   9. Anesthesia and analgesia (R)
   10. Other medications during labor, delivery, and puerperium (R)
   11. Forceps delivery (R)

12. Cesarean section and indications (R)

13. Identification abnormalities of placenta, cord, and amniotic fluid (R)

14. Identification of anemia (R)

15. Management of complications of labor and delivery (R)

16. Management of complications of anesthesia (R)

17. Performance of supplemental tests and procedures consistent with the diagnosis (e.g., cultures, coagulation studies, x-rays, pelvimetry, fetal monitoring, cord blood studies, etc.) (R)

18. Transfusions (R)

19. Identification of complications of puerperium (R)

20. Management of complications of puerperium (R)

21. Referrals, consultations, and reports (H,C)

22. Extended length of stay mother and/or infant (C,R)

23. Follow-up of abnormal laboratory findings (R)

24. Exchange transfusions (R)

25. Postpartum counseling on problems (H,C,R)

26. Newborn resuscitation (H,R)

27. Management of infant complications and morbidity (R)

28. Premature nursery care (R)

29. Infant intensive care (R)

30. Infant blood studies and procedures (R)

31. Follow-up of infant positive findings (R,C)

C. Postpartum

1. Identify complications of previous contraceptive use (R)

2. Identify abnormal menstrual history (R)

3. Identify abnormal history contraindicating the use of particular forms of contraception (R)

4. Identify and manage problems in perineal repair (R)

5. Treatment of abnormal conditions (e.g., vaginitis, cervicitis) (R)

6. Supplemental laboratory and other procedures consistent with the diagnosis (e.g., CBC or HB/Hct, WBC, and differential) (R)

7. Referrals (e.g., LaLeche League, other medical specialist, social worker, etc.) (R)

III. Maintenance of Health

A. Prenatal

1. Identification of patient with short pregnancy interval (R)

2. Evaluation of health and nutritional status prior to pregnancy (R)

3. Recording of height, weight, and dietary intake (P,R)

4. Identification of patient with allergy or drug sensitivity (R)

5. Identification of pre-existing medical, surgical, or dental disease (R)

6. Referral for management of concurrent medical, surgical, or dental disease (R)

7. Therapy for nausea and vomiting and other symptoms of pregnancy (R)

8. Preventive therapy for varicosities, striae, etc. (R)

9. Dietary supplements (R)

10. Recommended changes in dietary intake (R)

11. Counseling on daily activities during pregnancy (e.g., diet, exercise, sleep, employment, travel, bathing, etc.) (P,C,R)

12. Counseling on emotional adjustment to pregnancy (R)

13. Counseling in preparation for the baby (P,C,R)

14. Inquiry regarding the development of family or household problems relating to the birth of the infant (C,R)

B. Labor and Delivery
1. Management of postpartum depression and other psychiatric or social problems relating to the birth of the infant (R)

2. Appropriate referrals for management of above (R)

3. Same as 14 under prenatal

C. Postpartum
1. Identification of newly developed general medical and surgical problems (P,R)

2. Referral for management of the above (R)

3. Referral for general medical supervision (R)

4. Referral for well-baby care (P,C,R)

5. Same as 14 under prenatal

IV. Rehabilitation
As we have defined rehabilitation, it is an extension of minimization and these indicators address more specifically the definitive identification and management of multiple or extensive, often long-term conditions, including those in the socioenvironmental area.
A. Prenatal
1. Identification of sociodemographically high-risk pregnancy (e.g., unwed mother, teen-age pregnancy, grandmultipara, elderly primipara, etc.) (P,R)

2. Identification of individuals with serious medical or family problems (P,C,R)

3. Identification of mother or father who is drug addicted (R)

4. Identification of individuals exposed to environmental hazards or deprivation (P,C,R)

5. Management of above conditions or problems by provider (includes referrals and coordinative services) and by patient (C,R)

6. Inquiry regarding the development of health and socioenvironmental problems (P,C,R)

7. Emotional support for patients suffering a spontaneous abortion or other untoward early outcome of pregnancy (R)

8. Counseling and/or special arrangements for inappropriate utilization of services (e.g., chronic appointment breaking) (P,R)

B. Labor and Delivery
1. Identification of infants with congenital defects and other disabilities (R)

2. Management (including referral) of health, family, and social problems relating to above conditions (R)

3. Genetic counseling referrals (H,C,R)

4. Psychiatric and related services in instances of death of mother or infant (R)

5. Extended length of stay of mother or infant (R)

6. Management of mother and infant suffering from drug addiction (R)

7. Counseling and management of mother/infant relationship in cases of unwanted baby, mentally retarded mother, mother with serious physical disabilities, etc. (R)

8. Same as 6 under prenatal

C. Postpartum
1. Identification of family problems relating to sexual function and use of contraception (P,R)

2. Referral and continued management of serious problems of mother or infant (R)

3. Same as 6 under prenatal

V. Accessibility
A. Prenatal
1. Hours of program operation (P)

2. Eligibility requirements prenatal program (P,C)

3. Transportation to facilities, transit time, convenient location (P,C)

4. Method of payment and prepayment (P,C,H,R)

5. Patient financial data (C)

6. Patient occupational and educational data (R)

7. Program policies (C)

8. Mother's perceived comfort to questions re: maternity process, infant care, health, family and environmental problems (C)

9. Reason for selecting source of prenatal care (C)

B. Labor and Delivery

1. Method of payment, hospitalization (H)

2. Eligibility requirements, hospital (H)

3. Hospital policies (H)

4. Reaching hospital and/or M.D. when in labor (C)

5. Mother's perceived comfort to questions re: labor, delivery, and puerperium; maternal and infant care; health and family problems (C)

C. Postpartum

1-7. Same as under prenatal (P,C,H,R)

8. Mother's perceived comfort to questions re: family planning, infant and personal health, family and environmental problems (C)

9. Mother's awareness of sources of well-baby care (P,C)

10. Patient's environmental (household) characteristics (C)

VI. Availability

A. Prenatal

1. Sources of prenatal care (C)

2. Type of practice (P)

3. Type of staffing, classification professional personnel (P)

4. Staff available to counsel patients (C)

5. Type of referrals, community resources (P,C,R)

6. Volume of patients services, other service and patient population statistics (P)

7. Possibility of abortion (P)

B. Labor and Delivery

1. Type of hospital where delivered (H)

2. Hospitals utilized for delivery by program (H)

3. Number of delivery rooms (H)

4. Number of delivery rooms equipped for C-section (H)

5. Number of labor beds (H)

6. Number of maternity beds (H)

7. Number of bassinets (H)

8. Obstetrics recovery room (H)

9. Location blood and fibrinogen (H)

10. Transfer of newborns (H)

11. Categories of professional and nonprofessional staff (H)

12. Staff available to counsel patients (C)

13. Type of referrals, community resources (P,C,R)

14. Volume of deliveries and abortions and other service and patient population statistics (H)

C. Postpartum
   1. Sources of postpartum and interconceptional care (C)

   2-6. Same as 2-6 under prenatal (P,C,R)

VII. Adequacy
  A. Prenatal
   1. Routine and selective content of initial prenatal visit (P,R)

   2. Routine and selective content of subsequent prenatal visits (P,R)

   3. Continuity in source of prenatal care (C)

   4. Program awareness of other sources of care utilized by patient (C)

   5. Use of ACOG record forms (P)

   6. Referral forms and return reports (P)

   7. Prenatal abstract sent to hospital (P)

  B. Labor and Delivery
   1. Organization hospital department of obstetrics-gynecology (H)

   2. Continuity in source prenatal and delivery care (P,C)

   3. Place of delivery (R)

   4. Staff performing deliveries (H,R)

   5. Staff resuscitating newborn (H)

   6. Staff attending newborn (H,R)

   7. Physician in intensive care (H)

   8. Nursing/patient ratios — maternity, newborn, and intensive care services (H)

   9. Nursing staff delivery room by shift (H)

   10. Staff administering anesthesia (H,R)

   11. Staffing laboratory and x-ray service, including emergency procedures (H)

   12. Staff observing first hour after delivery (H)

13. Occupancy rate in maternity beds (H)
14. Percent obstetric patients having Hb/Hct (H)
15. Percent obstetric patients having urinalysis (H)
16. Infant resuscitation island in delivery room (H)
17. Ratio bassinets to maternity beds (H)
18. Exchange transfusion set-up (H)
19. Use of ACOG record forms (H)
20. Time to complete forms (H)

C. Postpartum
   1. Routine and selective content postpartum visit (P,C)
   2. Continuity in maternity and postpartum care (C)

VIII. Responsiveness
A. Prenatal
   1. Appointment system (P,C)
   2. Follow-up of broken appointments (P)
   3. Reason for not keeping appointments (C)
   4. Management of walk-ins (P)
   5. Waiting time (P,C)
   6. Coverage after hours (P)
   7. Physical setting (P,C)
   8. Privacy (P,C)
   9. Dignity of care (C)
   10. Perceived personalization of care (C)
   11. Certain (e.g., patient initiated) referrals and selective activities during prenatal visits particularly relating to socioenvironmental factors (P,R)
   12. Father's involvement prenatal visits and classes (P,C)
   13. Hospital tour (P,H,C)

B. Labor and Delivery
   1. Information regarding hospital's policies and practices (H)
   2. Visiting hours (H,C)
   3. Physical setting (H,C)
   4. Perceived personalization of care (C)
   5. Rooming-in, opportunities for mother/infant contact (H,C)
   6. Father's involvement labor and delivery (H,C,R)
   7. Discussion of anesthesia (H,C)

8. Referrals for management socioenvironmental problems and hazards (H,C,R)

9. Certain extended stays mother and/or infant (C,R)

C. Postpartum
   1. Follow-up of broken appointments (P)
   2. Desired and prescribed method of contraception (R)

IX. Effectiveness
A. Prenatal
   1. Planned or unplanned pregnancy (C,R)
   2. Reason for seeking care initially (C)
   3. Time of initiation of prenatal care (C,R)
   4. Appropriateness of source of care for early pregnancy (C)
   5. Broken appointments (C,R)
   6. Number of prenatal visits (R)
   7. Compliance with therapy and recommended modifications (P,C)
   8. Perceived change in health problem status (C)
   9. Duration of and limitation posed by health problem (C)
   10. Satisfaction with amount of information (C)
   11. Satisfaction with setting (C)
   12. Satisfaction with care received (C)
   13. Patient knowledge gestation and labor (C)
   14. Complications of pregnancy (R)

B. Labor and Delivery
   1. Mother's perception of labor, delivery, and anesthesia (C)
   2. Maternal and infant mortality (H,R)
   3. Maternal and infant complication relating to delivery (H,R)
   4. Complication and morbidity relating to the puerperium (H,R)
   5. Perineal repair and lacerations (H,R)
   6. Prematurity (H,R)
   7. Neonatal complications and morbidity (H,R)
   8. Prenatal/maternal mortality and morbidity committee or functional equivalent (H)
   9. Extended length of stay (C,R)
   10. Patient knowledge labor and delivery and infant care (C)
   11. Perceived health status of mother and infant in hospital (C)
   12. Satisfaction with setting (C)

13. Satisfaction with care received, desired changes (C)

C. Postpartum
   1. Status of smoking habit (C)
   2. Perceived maternal and infant health and developmental status and problems (C)
   3. Perceived socioenvironmental status and problems (C)
   4. Perceived child care confidence and problems (C)
   5. Perceived improvement in above problems (C)
   6. Appropriateness of patient's source of care for problems (C)
   7. Knowledge and understanding of physician assessment maternal and infant health status and problems (C)
   8. Return for postpartum visit (P,C)
   9. Return for continued interconceptional care (P,C)
   10. Use of family planning (C,R)
   11. Keeping appointment for well-baby care (P,C)

Author Index

Subject Index

About the Author

Dr. Avedis Donabedian maintains a longtime association with the University of Michigan where he is pres-
ently the Nathan Sinai Distinguished Professor of Public
Health. Dr. Donabedian, who received his M.D. from
the American University of Beirut and M.P.H. from the
Harvard School of Public Health, taught previously at
the American University of Beirut, at the Harvard
School of Public Health and at New York Medical College. Dr. Donabedian was elected a member of The In-
stitute of Medicine, National Academy of Sciences in
1971. The author of numerous books and articles, his
most recent text was *Benefits in Medical Care Programs.*
His previous publications have won the DEAN CON-
LEY Award of the American College of Hospital
Administrators in 1969, the NORMAN A. WELCH
Award of the National Association of Blue Shield Plans
in 1976, and the ELIZUR WRIGHT Award of the
American Risk and Insurance Association in 1978.